MCQ IN PHARMACOLOGY

Mohd Farook
M.Pharma (Pharmaceutical Chemistry)
M.A.Sociology, **PGDCA**

Published by CreateSpace Independent Publisheing Platform

First Edition

Medical & Pharmacy are fast growing professions with a wide range of opportunities open to the students after a basic degree. These professions play a vital role in health health care management.

This book will be of immense value for students to develop themselves as the meritorious & motivated candidates for admission to post graduate courses like M.D., M.S.& M.Pharma.

I compliment the author for his pains-taking efforts in mobilizing a very large number of good MCQs from a vast subject like Pharmacology. Adequate coverage of of all topics is done.

I feel that this book will be a very useful companion for professional PG entrence exams.

Mr. Ashish Pathak
Asst. Professor
Department of Pharmaceutical Chemistry
Ravishankar College of Pharmacy Bhopal

Acknowledgments

I acknowledge the help rendered by the following well-wishers during the preparation of the manuscript.

Mr. Ashish Pathak
Asst. Professor
Department of Pharmaceutical Chemistry
Ravishankar College of Pharmacy Bhopal

Mr. Deep Chand Mudiya
Senior Research Officer
Department of Pharmaceutical Chemistry
Sapience Bio Anlaytical Research Lab Bhopal

Mr. Himanshu Basrani
Nephrology Scientific Buisness officer
Dr. Reddy's Laboratories

Ms. Nida Khan
Asst. Professor
Department of Pharmaceutical Chemistry
Ravishankar College of Pharmacy Bhopal

Finally, I would like to place on record the generous help rendered by
Create Space Independent Publishing Platform
In bringing out this book

-Mohd .Farook

Content

1. Introduction to Pharmacology: Basic Principal

1. Pharmacokinetics is:
a) The study of biological and therapeutic effects of drugs
b) The study of absorption, distribution, metabolism and excretion of drugs
c) The study of mechanisms of drug action
d) The study of methods of new drug development

2. What does "pharmacokinetics" include?
a) Pharmacological effects of drugs
b) Unwanted effects of drugs
c) Chemical structure of a medicinal agent
d) Distribution of drugs in the organism

3. What does "pharmacokinetics" include?
a) Localization of drug action
b) Mechanisms of drug action
c) Excretion of substances
d) Interaction of substances

4. The main mechanism of most drugs absorption in GI tract is:
a) Active transport (carrier-mediated diffusion)
b) Filtration (aqueous diffusion)
c) Endocytosis and exocytosis
d) Passive diffusion (lipid diffusion)

5. What kind of substances can't permeate membranes by passive diffusion?
a) Lipid-soluble
b) Non-ionized substances
c) Hydrophobic substances
d) Hydrophilic substances

6. A hydrophilic medicinal agent has the following property:
a) Low ability to penetrate through the cell membrane lipids
b) Penetrate through membranes by means of endocytosis

c) Easy permeation through the blood-brain barrier
d) High reabsorption in renal tubules

7. What is implied by «active transport»?
a) Transport of drugs trough a membrane by means of diffusion
b) Transport without energy consumption
c) Engulf of drug by a cell membrane with a new vesicle formation
d) Transport against concentration gradient

8. What does the term "bioavailability" mean?
a) Plasma protein binding degree of substance
b) Permeability through the brain-blood barrier
c) Fraction of an uncharged drug reaching the systemic circulation following any route administration
d) Amount of a substance in urine relative to the initial doze

9. The reasons determing bioavailability are:
a) Rheological parameters of blood
b) Amount of a substance obtained orally and quantity of intakes
c) Extent of absorption and hepatic first-pass effect
d) Glomerular filtration rate

10. Which route of drug administration is most likely to lead to the first-pass effect?
a) Sublingual
b) Oral
c) Intravenous
d) Intramuscular

11. What is characteristic of the oral route?
a) Fast onset of effect
b) Absorption depends on GI tract secretion and motor function
c) A drug reaches the blood passing the liver
d) The sterilization of medicinal forms is obligatory

12. Tick the feature of the sublingual route:
a) Pretty fast absorption
b) A drug is exposed to gastric secretion
c) A drug is exposed more prominent liver metabolism
d) A drug can be administrated in a variety of doses

13. Pick out the parenteral route of medicinal agent administration:

a) Rectal
b) Oral
c) Sublingual
d) Inhalation

14. Parenteral administration:
a) Cannot be used with unconsciousness patients
b) Generally results in a less accurate dosage than oral administration
c) Usually produces a more rapid response than oral administration
d) Is too slow for emergency use

15. What is characteristic of the intramuscular route of drug administration?
a) Only water solutions can be injected
b) Oily solutions can be injected
c) Opportunity of hypertonic solution injections
d) The action develops slower, than at oral administration

16. All of the following statements about efficacy and potency are true EXCEPT:
a) Efficacy is usually a more important clinical consideration than potency
b) Efficacy is the maximum effect of a drug
c) Potency is a comparative measure, refers to the different doses of two drugs that are needed to produce the same effect
d) The ED $_{50}$ is a measure of drug's efficacy

17. Give the definition for a therapeutical dose:
a) The amount of a substance to produce the minimal biological effect
b) The amount of a substance to produce effects hazardous for an organism
c) The amount of a substance to produce the required effect in most patients
d) The amount of a substance to accelerate an increase of concentration of medicine in an organism

18. Pick out the correct definition of a toxic dose:
a) The amount of substance to produce the minimal biological effect
b) The amount of substance to produce effects hazardous for an organism
c) The amount of substance to produce the necessary effect in most of patients
d) The amount of substance to fast creation of high concentration of medicine in
an organism

19. Which effect may lead to toxic reactions when a drug is taken continuously or repeatedly?
a) Refractoriness
b) Cumulative effect
c) Tolerance
d) Tachyphylaxis

20. What term is used to describe a more gradual decrease in responsiveness to a drug, taking days or weeks to develop?
a) Refractorines
b) Cumulative effect
c) Tolerance
d) Tachyphylaxis

21. What term is used to describe a decrease in responsiveness to a drug which develops in a few minutes?
a) Refractoriness
b) Cumulative effect
c) Tolerance
d) Tachyphylaxis

22. Tachyphylaxis is:
a) A drug interaction between two similar types of drugs
b) Very rapidly developing tolerance
c) A decrease in responsiveness to a drug, taking days or weeks to develop
d) None of the above

23. Tolerance and drug resistance can be a consequence of:
a) Drug dependence
b) Increased metabolic degradation
c) Depressed renal drug excretion
d) Activation of a drug after hepatic first-pass

24. Tolerance and drug resistance can be a consequence of:
a) Change in receptors, loss of them or exhaustion of mediators
b) Increased receptor sensitivity
c) Decreased metabolic degradation
d) Decreased renal tubular secretion

25. Tolerance develops because of:
a) Diminished absorption
b) Rapid excretion of a drug
c) Both of the above
d) None of the above

26. The situation when failure to continue administering the drug results in serious psychological and somatic disturbances is called?
a) Tachyphylaxis
b) Sensibilization
c) Abstinence syndrome
d) Idiosyncrasy

27. What is the type of drug-to-drug interaction which is connected with processes of absorption, biotransformation,distribution and excretion?
a) Pharmacodynamic interaction
b) Physical and chemical interaction
c) Pharmaceutical interaction
d) Pharmacokinetic interaction

28. What is the type of drug-to-drug interaction which is the result of interaction at receptor, cell, enzyme or organ level?
a) Pharmacodynamic interaction
b) Physical and chemical interaction
c) Pharmaceutical interaction
d) Pharmacokinetic interaction

29. What phenomenon can occur in case of using a combination of drugs?
a) Tolerance
b) Tachyphylaxis
c) Accumulation
d) Synergism

30. If two drugs with the same effect, taken together, produce an effect that is equal in magnitude to the sum of the effects of the drugs given individually, it is called as:
a) Antagonism
b) Potentiation
c) Additive effect
d) None of the above

31. What does the term "potentiation" mean?
a) Cumulative ability of a drug
b) Hypersensitivity to a drug
c) Fast tolerance developing
d) Intensive increase of drug effects due to their combination

32. The types of antagonism are:
a) Summarized
b) Potentiated
c) Additive
d) Competitive

33. The term "chemical antagonism" means that:
a) two drugs combine with one another to form an inactive compound
b) two drugs combine with one another to form a more active compound
c) two drugs combine with one another to form a more water soluble compound
d) two drugs combine with one another to form a more fat soluble compound

34. A teratogenic action is:
a) Toxic action on the liver
b) Negative action on the fetus causing fetal malformation
c) Toxic action on blood system
d) Toxic action on kidneys

35. Characteristic unwanted reaction which isn't related to a dose or to a pharmacodynamic property of a drug is called:
a) Idiosyncrasy
b) Hypersensitivity
c) Tolerance
d) Teratogenic action

36. Idiosyncratic reaction of a drug is:
a) A type of hypersensitivity reaction
b) A type of drug antagonism
c) Unpredictable, inherent, qualitatively abnormal reaction to a drug
d) Quantitatively exaggerated response

37. Therapeutic index (TI) is:
a) A ratio used to evaluate the safety and usefulness of a drug for indication
b) A ratio used to evaluate the effectiveness of a drug
c) A ratio used to evaluate the bioavailability of a drug
d) A ratio used to evaluate the elimination of a drug

38. Which of the following is NOT part of the etymology of the word pharmacology?
a) Medicine
b) Drug
c) Herb
d) Poison

39. Which of the following describes an agonist?
a) Any substance that brings about a change in biologic function through its chemical action
b) A specific regulatory molecule in the biologic system where a drug interacts
c) A drug that binds to a receptor and stimulates cellular activity
d) A drug that binds to a receptor and inhibits or opposes cellular activity

40.Xenobiotics are considered:
a) Endogenous
b) Exogenous
c) Inorganic poisons
d) Toxins

41. Which of the following would be a toxin (poison of biological origin)?
a) Pb
b) As
c) Hg
d) Atropine

42. The vast majority of drugs have molecular weights (MW) between 100 and 1,000.Large drugs, such as alteplase (t-PA), must be administered:
a) Into the compartment where they have their effect
b) Orally so they do not absorb too quickly
c) Rectally to prevent irritation to the stomach lining and vessels
d) Via the intraosseous (IO) route

43. Which of the following occurs with drugs that are extremely small, such as Lithium?
a) Receptor mediated endocytosis
b) Minor drug movement within the body
c) Vasodilation when injected intravenously (IV)
d) Specific receptor binding
e) Nonspecific binding

44. Drugs fit receptors using the lock and key model. Covalent bonds are the ____ and the ____ specific.
a) Strongest; Most
b) Strongest; Least
c) Weakest; Most
d) Weakest; Least

45. Warfarin (Coumadin) is given as a racemic mixture with the S enantiomer being four times more active than the R enantiomer. If the mixture of Warfarin given is 50% S and 50% R, what is the potency compared with a 100% R enantiomer solution?
a) $4 * R + 1 * S = 1$
b) $4 * R + 1 * S = 1.5$
c) $4 * R + 1 * S = 2$
d) $4 * R + 1 * S = 2.5$
e) $4 * R + 1 * S = 4$

46. What determines the degree of movement of a drug between body compartments?
a) Partition constant
b) Degree of ionization
c) pH
d) Size
e) All of the above

47. Which of the following is NOT a protein target for drug binding?
a) Side of action (transport)
b) Enzymes
c) Carrier molecules
d) Receptors
e) Ion channels

48. Which of the following is an example of a drug acting directly through receptors?
a) Protamine binds stoichiometrically to heparin anticoagulants
b) Adrenergic beta blockers for thyroid hormone-induced tachycardia
c) Epinephrine for increasing heart rate and blood pressure
d) Cancer chemotherapeutic agents

49. What is added with drug subclassification, such as an antitubercular drug versus an antibacterial drug?
a) Cost
b) Size
c) Ionization
d) Precision

50. What type of drug is propranolol (Inderal)?
a) Anticonvulsive
b) Antihypertensive
c) Antinauseant

51.Which of the following is considered the brand name?
a) Propranolol
b) Inderal
c) Adrenergic ß-blocker
d) "off label" use

52.Which of the following is considered the class?
a) Propranolol
b) Inderal
c) Adrenergic ß-blocker
d) "off label" use

53. Which of the following cases would be contraindicated for propranolol (Inderal)?
a) Hypertension
b) Essential tremor
c) Angina
d) Asthma

54. Which of the following adverse effects (side-effects) is NOT commonly seen with cholinergic antagonists?
a) Blurred vision
b) Confusion
c) Miosis
d) Constipation

55.The drug chloramphenicol (Chloromycetin) is risky for which of the following?
a) Neonates
b) Geriatric patients
c) Adult males
d) Obese patients

56.How does the glomerular filtration rate (GFR) change after the age of 40?
a) Increase 1% each year
b) Increases 2% each year
c) Decreases 1% each year
d) Decreases 2% each year

57. A decrease in renal and liver function, as seen in the elderly, would pro-long drug half-life, _____ plasma protein binding, and _____ volume of distribution.
a) Increase; Increase
b) Decrease; Decrease
c) Increase; Decrease
d) Decrease; Increase

58. When prescribing isoniazid (Rimifon), pharmacogenetics must be considered as >90% of Asians and certain other groups are _____ acetylators, and thus have a _____ blood concentration of a given dose and a decreased risk of toxicity.
a) Slow; Increased
b) Slow; Decreased
c) Fast; Increased
d) Fast; Decrease

59. Which of the following are the two modifying factors that contribute to why women have higher blood peak concentrations of alcohol than men when consuming equivalent amounts?
a) Lower blood volume & increased hormones
b) Lower fat content & more gastric alcohol dehydrogenase (ADH)
c) Higher fat content & more gastric alcohol dehydrogenase (ADH)
d) Higher fat content & less gastric alcohol dehydrogenase (ADH)

Answer Key

01-B 02-D 03-C 04-D 05-D 06-A 07-D 08-C 09-C 10-B 11-B 12-A 13-D 14-C 15-B 16-D 17-C 18-B 19-B 19-B 21-D 22-B 23-B 24-A 25-D 26-C 27-D 28-A 29-D 30-C 31-D 32-D 33-A 34-B 35-B 36-C 37-A 38-C 39-C 40-C 41-D 42-A 43-E 44-B 45-D 46-C 47-A 48-C 49-D 50-B 51-B 52-C 53-D 54-C 55-A 56-C 57-B 58-D 59-D

1.2 Pharmacokinetic Basics

1. Which of the following would receive drug slowly?
a) Liver
b) Brain
c) Fat
d) Muscle

2. Which of the following is the least important for passage through capillary walls but the most important for passage through the cell wall?
a) Molecular size

b) Lipid solubility
c) Diffusion constant
d) pH

3. Which of the following is the most important for movement through capillary walls?
a) Molecular size
b) Lipid solubility
c) Diffusion constant
d) pH

4. Which of the following locations would most trap a lipid soluble drug?
a) Blood
b) Intestines
c) Brain
d) Stomach

5. What type of drugs can cross the blood-brain barrier (BBB)?
a) Large and lipid-soluble
b) Large and lipid-insoluble
c) Small and lipid-soluble
d) Small and lipid-insoluble

6.Acidic drugs, such as phenytoin, bind primarily to which of the following plasma proteins?
a) ál-fetoprotein (AFP)
b) GC Globulin
c) Albumin
d) ál-acid glycoprotein (AAG)

7. Basic drugs, such as lidocaine, bind primarily to which of the following plasma proteins?
a) alpha1-fetoprotein (AFP)
b) Gc-Globulin (GcG)
c) Albumin
d) alpha 1-acid glycoprotein (AAG)

8. A decrease in drug-protein binding will lead to which of the following?
a) Decrease in the unbound drug concentration
b) Increase in free drug
c) Increase in rate of drug elimination
d) Decrease in volume of distribution

9. A patient presents with acute-onset cirrhosis of the liver. They are found to have hypoalbuminemia. In severe cirrhosis it is expected that AAG will be decreased, but the patient presents with increased AAG due to the inflammatory response. Which of the following is the most likely?
a) Increased acidic drug binding and increased basic drug binding
b) Increased acidic drug binding and decreased basic drug binding
c) Decreased acidic drug binding and increased basic drug binding
d) Decreased acidic drug binding and decreased basic drug binding

10. Which of the following is NOT a site of loss (where drug is not used)?
a) Fat
b) GI tract
c) Muscle
d) Site lacking receptors

11. Which of the following locations can accumulate lipid-soluble drugs, has little or no receptors, and can hold distributed drugs like barbiturates?
a) Liver
b) Kidney
c) Brain
d) Fat

12. Which of the following locations has high blood flow and is a site of excretion?
a) Liver
b) Kidney
c) Brain
d) Fat

13. Which of the following can be treated with drugs due to a leaky area in the blood-brain barrier near the medulla?
a) Seizures
b) Shivers
c) Diarrhea
d) Vomiting

14. What is the approximate lag time for equilibration between maternal blood and fetal tissues?
a) 20 mins
b) 40 mins
c) 1 hour
d) 2 hours

15. If protein plasma binding is decreased, how will volume of distribution be affected?

a) Increased

b) Decreased

c) Not changed

16. 400 mg of a drug is administered to a patient and the drug is later measured in plasma to be 1 μg/ml. What is the apparent volume of distribution (Vd)?

a) 0.04 L

b) 0.4 L

c) 4 L

d) 400 L

17. Elderly patients often have _____ muscle mass and thus a(n) _____ Vd.

a) More; Increased

b) More; Decreased

c) Less; Increased

d) Less; Decreased

18. Patients with ascites or edema would have _____ Vd for hydrophilic drugs, such as gentamicin.

a) Increased

b) Decreased

c) Unchanged

d) Unknown

Answer Key

1-C 2-B 3-A 4-D 5-C 6-C 7-D 8-C 9-C 10-C 11-D 12-B 13-D 14-B 15-A 16-D 17-D 18-A

1.3 Pharmacokinetic Principles: Absorption

1. Bioavailability (F) is the fraction or percentage of administered drug that reaches the systemic circulation via a given route as compared to what route?

a) Oral

b) IV (intravenous)

c) IO (intraosseous)

d) CSF (cerebrospinal fluid)

2. What organ is responsible for metabolism in the "first pass effect"?
a) Brain
b) Heart
c) Kidney
d) Liver

3. A patient is in the hospital and is stable on digoxin 0.175 mg IV qd (daily). How much digoxin in mg. would you need to give your patient orally, given that the bioavailability for oral digoxin tablets is 0.7?
a) $(0.175 * 0.7) / (1.0) = 0.1225$ mg
b) $(0.175 * 1) / (0.7) = 0.25$ mg
c) $(0.175 + 0.7) / (1.0) = 0.875$ mg
d) $(0.175 + 1) / (0.7) = 1.67$ mg

4. Given a graph of plasma drug concentration versus time, what part of the graph would be used to calculate bioavailability for a PO (oral) drug administration?
a) Maximum concentration
b) Steady concentration
c) Derivative of the curve (slope)
d) Integral of the curve (area underneath)

5. Which of the following routes of administration has a bioavailability of about 80-100%, is usually very slow absorbing, and has prolonged duration of action?
a) IV (intravenous)
b) IM (intramuscular)
c) SQ (subcutaneous)
d) Transdermal

6.Which of the following routers of administration is the most convenient, although may have a bioavailability anywhere from 5-100%?
a) PO (oral)
b) IV (intravenous)
c) IM (intramuscular)
d) SQ (subcutaneous)

7.Which of the following enteral administration routes has the largest first-pass effect?

a) SL (sublingual)
b) Buccal
c) Rectal
d) Oral

8.Epithelial cells are connected by ____, which are tough to cross and materials oftenmust pass through the cells. Endothelial cells of blood vessels are connected by ____,which proteins cannot cross but smaller drugs (MW 200-500) can.

a) Macular gap junctions; Tight junctions

b) Tight junctions; Macular gap junctions

c) Adherens junctions; Tight junctions

d) Tight junctions; Adherens junctions

e) Macular gap junctions; Adherens junctions

9. 400 mg of a drug is administered to a patient and the drug is later measured in plasma to be 1 μg/ml. What is the apparent volume of distribution (Vd)?
a) 0.04 L
b) 0.4 L
c) 40 L
d) 400 L

10. Elderly patients often have ____ muscle mass and thus a(n) ____ Vd.
a) More; Increased
b) More; Decreased
c) Less; Increased
d) Less; Decreased

11. Patients with ascites or edema would have ____ Vd for hydrophilic drugs, such asgentamicin.
a) Increased
b) Decreased
c) Unchanged

Answer Key

1-B 2-D 3-B 4-D 5-D 6-A 7-D 8-B 9-D 10-D 11-A

1.4 Pharmacokinetic Principles: Drug Movement

1. Pharmacokinetics is the effect of the _____ and pharmacodynamics is the effect of the_____.
a) Drug on a drug; Body on the drug
b) Body on the drug; Drug on a drug
c) Drug on the body; Body on the drug
d) Body on the drug; Drug on the body
e) Drug on a drug; Drug on a drug

2. Which of the following is NOT an action of the body on a drug?
a) Absorption
b) Distribution
c) Metabolism
d) Excretion
e) Side effects

3. If a drug is 80% bound to blood elements or plasma proteins, what part is considered the free form?
a) 20%
b) 40%
c) 50%
d) 80%

4. Which of the following describes minimal effective concentration (MEC)?
a) The minimal drug plasma concentration that can be detected
b) The minimal drug plasma concentration to enter tissues
c) The minimal drug plasma concentration to interact with receptors
d) The minimal drug plasma concentration to produce effect

5. If a patient misses three doses of their daily drug, which of the following (in general) is the best solution?
a) Take a 4x dose at the next dose time
b) Wait 3 more days (week total) then return to normal regimen
c) Do nothing and continue normal regimen
d) Setup an appointment to have the patient evaluated

6. Which of the following drug permeation mechanisms involves polar substances too large to enter cells by other means, such as iron or vitamin B12?
a) Aqueous diffusion
b) Lipid diffusion
c) Carrier molecules
d) Endocytosis and exocytosis

7. Which of the following drug permeation mechanisms occurs across epithelial tight junctions and is driven by a concentration gradient?

a) Aqueous diffusion
b) Lipid diffusion
c) Carrier molecules
d) Endocytosis and exocytosis

8. Which of the following drug permeation mechanisms uses the Henderson-Hasselbalch equation for the ratio of solubility for the weak acid or weak base?
a) Aqueous diffusion
b) Lipid diffusion
c) Carrier molecules
d) Endocytosis and exocytosis

9. Which of the following drug permeation mechanisms is used for peptides, amino acids, glucose, and other large or insoluble molecules?
a) Aqueous diffusion
b) Lipid diffusion
c) Carrier molecules
d) Endocytosis and exocytosis

10.Which of the following drug permeation mechanisms uses caveolae?
a) Aqueous diffusion
b) Lipid diffusion
c) Carrier molecules
d) Endocytosis and exocytosis

11. Using the Fick Law of Diffusion, how will flux change if membrane thickness is doubled?
a) It will double
b) It will quadruple
c) It will halve
d) It will quarter

12. Using the Fick Law of Diffusion, how will flux change if the permeability coefficient is quadrupled?
a) It will double
b) It will quadruple
c) It will halve
d) It will quarter

13. Which of the following is the amount of a drug absorbed per the amount administered?

a) Bioavailability

b) Bioequivalence

c) Drug absorption

d) Bioinequivalence

14.Which of the following is NOT needed for drug bioequivalence?

a) Same active ingredients

b) Same strength or concentration

c) Same dosage form

d) Same route of administration

e) Same side effects

15.For intravenous (IV) dosages, what is the bioavailability assumed to be?

a) 25%

b) 50%

c) 75%

d) 100%

16. Although morphine (Avinza, Oramorph SR, MS Contin) is well-absorbed when administered orally (PO), how much of the drug is metabolized on its first pass through the liver?

a) 90%

b) 70%

c) 50%

d) 30%

17. For a generic drug to be bioequivalent to an innovator drug (per FDA), it must be measured in _____ of subjects to fall within _____ of the mean of the test population bioavailability.

a) 50; 50

b) 80; 20

c) 20; 80

d) 95; 5

18. Using the FDA bioequivalence rule, how much variation could a generic drug Potentially have from an innovator and still be considered equivalent?

a) 100%

b) 20%

c) 40%

d) 60%

19. Which of the following is NOT a pharmacokinetic process?
a) Alteration of the drug by liver enzymes
b) Drug metabolites are removed in the urine
c) Movement of drug from the gut into general circulation
d) The drug causes dilation of coronary vessels

20. Which of the following can produce a therapeutic response? A drug that is:
a) Bound to plasma albumin
b) Concentrated in the bile
c) Concentrated in the urine
d) Unbound to plasma proteins

21. Which of the following most correctly describes steroid hormones with respect to their ability to gain access to intracellular binding sites?
a) They cross the cell membrane via aqueous pores
b) They have a high permeability coefficient
c) They are passively transported via membrane carriers
d) They require vesicular transport

Answer Key

1-B 2-E 3-A 4-D 5-C 6-D 7-A 8-B 9-C 10-D 11-C 12-B 13-A 14-E 15-D 16-A 17-B 18-C 19-D 20-D 21-B

1.5 Pharmacokinetic Principles: pH and Drug Movement

1 . Most drugs are either _____ acids or _____ bases.
a) Strong; Strong
b) Strong; Weak
c) Weak; Weak
d) Weak; Strong

2. Aspirin readily donates a proton in aqueous solutions and pyrimethamine readily accepts a proton in aqueous solution. Thus, aspirin is a(b) _____ and pyrimethamine is a(n) _____.
a) Acid; Base
b) Base; Acid
c) Acid; Acid
d) Base; Base

3.Given the equilibrium HA <=> A- + H+ (acid) and BH+ <=> B + H+ (base), in an acid environment (low pH) the acid reaction will move to the _____ and the base reaction will move to the _____.

a) Right; Left
b) Right; Right
c) Left; Right
d) Left; Left

4. What form of a drug is more lipid-soluble, and thus would remain trapped within a compartment where the pH does not favor the lipid-soluble form?
a) Strong acid (A-)
b) Weak acid (A-)
c) Neutral (AH and B)
d) Weak base (BH+)

5. The lipid-soluble form of a base is _____ and the lipid-soluble form of an acid is_____.
a) Protonated; Protonated
b) Protonated; Unprotonated
c) Unprotonated; Unprotonated
d) Unprotonated; Protonated

6. If the pKa of Aspirin (acetylsalicylic acid) is 3.5 and the pH of the stomach is 2.5,how much Aspirin is in the protonated species in the stomach and is this the amount available for absorption?
a) $\approx$ 91%; Yes
b) $\approx$ 91%; No
c) $\approx$ 9%; Yes
d) $\approx$ 9%; No

7. What percentage of Aspirin would be ionized in the blood compartment (pH = 7.4) assuming pH is 7.5 and Aspirin pKa is 3.5?
a) $(10,000 - 1) / 1 = 99.99\%$
b) $(100 - 1) / 1 = 99\%$
c) None
d) $1 / (100 - 1) = 0.9\%$

8. If the pH - pKa = -1, what percentage of weak base is nonionized?
a) 99
b) 90
c) 50
d) 10

9. If the pH - pka = 2, what percentage of weak acid is nonionized?
a) 99
b) 90
c) 50
d) 1

10. If pH > pKa, the drug is ____ and if pH < pKa, the drug is ____. An unprotonated acid is ____ and a protonated base is ____.
a) Protonated; Unprotonated; Charged; Charged
b) Protonated; Unprotonated; Neutral; Neutral
c) Unprotonated; Protonated; Charged; Charged
d) Unprotonated; Protonated; Neutral; Charged

11. Weak acids are excreted faster in ____ urine and weak bases are excreted faster in____ urine.
a) Acidic; Alkaline
b) Alkaline; Acidic
c) Acidic; Neutral
d) Neutral; Alkaline

12. A patient presents with an overdose of acidic Aspirin. The drug ____ can be given to ____ the pH of the urine and trap the Aspirin, preventing further metabolism.
a) NaHCO3; Increase
b) NaHCO3; Decrease
c) NH4Cl; Increase
d) NH4Cl; Decrease

13. A patient presents with an overdose of alkaline Codeine. The drug ____ can be given to ____ the pH of the urine and trap the Codeine, preventing further metabolism.
a) NaHCO3; Increase
b) NaHCO3; Decrease
c) NH4Cl; Increase
d) NH4Cl; Decrease

14. The principle of drug manipulation for excretion of a drug out of the renal tubule can be accomplished by:
a) Acidifying the urinary pH
b) Adjusting the urinary pH to protonate weakly acidic drugs
c) Adjusting the urinary pH to unprotonate weakly basic drugs
d) Adjusting the urinary pH to ionize the drug

15.Aspirin is a weak organic acid with a pKa of 3.5. What percentage of a given dose will be in the lipid-soluble form at a stomach pH of 1.5?

a) About 1%

b) About 10%

c) About 50%

d) About 99%

16. For which of the following drugs is excretion most significantly accelerated by acidification of the urine?

a) Weak acid with pKa of 5.5

b) Weak acid with pKa of 3.5

c) Weak base with pKa of 7.5

d) Weak base with pKa of 7.1

17. A patient diagnosed with type 2 diabetes is administered an oral dose of 0.1 mg chloropropamide, an insulin secretagogue and weak acid with a pKa of 5.0. What is the amount of this drug that could be absorbed from the stomach at pH 2.0?

a) 99.9 µg

b) 90 µg

c) 50 µg

d) 0.05 mg

Answer Key

1-C 2-A 3-D 4-C 5-D 6-A 7-A 8-D 9-D 10-C 11-B 12-A 13-D 14-D 15-D 16-C 17-A

1.6 Pharmacokinetics: Drug Metabolism

1. Which of the following locations is the most likely for finding a free, unaltered drug?

a) Urine

b) Feces

c) Breast milk

d) Fat

2. Most drugs are active in their _____ form and inactive in their _____ form.

a) Non-polar; Polar

b) Polar; Non-polar

c) Water-soluble; Lipid-soluble

d) Lipid-insoluble; Water-insoluble

e) Neutral; Neutral

3. Drug biotransformation phase I makes drugs ____ polar for metabolism and phase II makes drugs ____ polar for excretion.
a) More; More
b) More; Less
c) Less; More
d) Less; Less

4. Which of the following is NOT a phase II substrate?
a) Glucuronic acid
b) Sulfuric acid
c) Acetic acid
d) Alcohol

5. Which of the following reactions is phase II and NOT phase I?
a) Oxidations
b) Reductions
c) Conjugations
d) Deaminations

6.Which of the following metabolically active tissues is the principle organ for drug metabolism?
a) Skin
b) Kidneys
c) Lungs
d) Liver

7. Damage at which of the following locations would most affect the goals of phase II biotransformation?
a) Skin
b) Kidneys
c) Lungs
d) Liver

8. What is the goal of the P450 system (microsomes pinched off from endoplasmic reticulum)?
a) Metabolism of substances
b) Detoxification of substances
c) Increasing pH of compartments containing substances
d) A & B

9. Regarding the microsomal drug metabolizing system, a patient with late stage alcoholism and liver damage would have more ETOH available due to which of the following concepts?

a) Increased induction
b) Decreased induction
c) Increased inhibition
d) Decreased inhibition

10.Regarding the microsomal drug metabolizing system, a patient who is a chronic user of barbiturates would need more drug to produce the same effects due to which of the following concepts?

a) Increased induction
b) Decreased induction
c) Increased inhibition
d) Decreased inhibition

11. Which of the following are the drugs that induce CYP 1A2 and the drugs that have their metabolism induced by 1A2?

a) Carbamazepine & phenobarbitol; Theophyline & warfarin
b) Phenobarbitol & phenytoin ; Phenytoin & warfarin
c) Carbamazepine & phenytoin; Warfarin
d) Carbamazepine; Cyclosporine

12. Which of the following are the drugs that inhibit CYP 1A2 and the drugs that have their metabolism inhibited by 1A2?

a) SSRIs; Phenytoin & warfarin
b) Amiodarone & cimetidine; Phenytoin & warfarin
c) Cimetidine, erythromycin, & grapefruit juice; Theophyline & warfarin
d) Cimetidine & erythromycin; Cyclosporine

13. Which of the following groups of people is the least likely to have bio-transformation effects due to altered hepatic function?

a) Infants
b) Adults
c) Elderly
d) Chronic alcoholics

14. In what location does amino acid conjugation of glycine (e.g. salicyclic acid) take place?

a) Microsomal
b) Cytosol
c) Mitochondria

15. Where does acetylation conjugation (e.g. isoniazid) and sulfate conjugation (e.g.acetaminophen) take place?

a) Microsomal

b) Cytosol

c) Mitochondria

16. Where does glucuronide conjucation (e.g. digoxin, bilirubin) take place?

a) Microsomal

b) Cytosol

c) Mitochondria

17.What is a result of conjugation of isoniazid via N-acetylation?

a) Detoxification of liver

b) Detoxification of kidneys

c) Detoxification of blood

d) Hepatotoxicity

Answer Key

1-D 2-A 3-A 4-D 5-C 6-D 7-B 8-D 9-D 10-A 11-A 12-C 13-B 14-C 15-B 16-A 17-D

1.7 Pharmacokinetics: Principles of Eliminations

1. One liter contains 1,000 mg of a drug. After one hour, 900 mg of the drug remains. What is the clearance?

a) 100 mL

b) 100 mL/hr

c) 1 mg/ml

d) 100 mg

2. To maintain a drug concentration at steady state, the dosing rate should equal the elimination rate. Which of the following is true? (CL = Drug Clearance)

a) Dosing rate = CL + target concentration

b) Dosing rate = CL - target concentration

c) Dosing rate = CL * target concentration

d) Dosing rate = CL / target concentration

3. Which of the following is most useful in determining the rate of elimination of a drug, in general?
a) Drug concentration in urine (renal elimination)
b) Drug concentration in stool (bilary elimination)
c) Drug concentration in blood
d) Drug concentration in brain

4. For first-order drug elimination, half-life t(1/2) is _____ at two places on the curve and a constant _____ is lost per unit time.
a) Equal; Amount
b) Equal; Percentage
c) Not equal; Amount
d) Not equal; Percentage

5. For first-order drug elimination, given the half-life equation of t(1/2) = (0.693 * Vd) / CL, how many half-lives would be necessary to reach steady state (≈95%) without a loading dose?
a) 1 to 2
b) 2 to 3
c) 3 to 4
d) 4 to 5

6. Which of the following is NOT a drug exhibiting zero-order elimination kinetics?
a) Aspirin
b) Morphine
c) Phenytoin
d) ETOH

7. For zero-order drug elimination, half-life t(1/2) is _____ at two places on the curve and a constant _____ is lost per unit time.
a) Equal; Amount
b) Equal; Percentage
c) Not equal; Amount
d) Not equal; Percentage

8. If a drug with a 2-hour half life is given with an initial dose of 8 mcg/ml, assuming first-order kinetics, how much drug will be left at 6 hours?
a) 8 mcg/ml
b) 4 mcg/ml
c) 2 mcg/ml
d) 1 mcg/ml

9. What are the units for steady-state concentration (Css), or infusion rate over

clearance?
a) mg/min
b) ml/min
c) mg/ml
d) ml/mg

10.What percentage of the steady-state drug concentration is achieved at 3.3 * t(1/2)?
a) 10%
b) 25%
c) 50%
d) 90%

10. Which of the following drugs would most likely need a loading dose to help reach therapeutic levels?
a) Acetaminophen, t(1/2) = 2 h
b) Aspirin, t(1/2) = 15 m
c) Tetracycline, t(1/2) = 11 h
d) Digitoxin, t(1/2) = 161 h

11. A target concentration of 7.5 mg/L of theophylline is required for a 60 kg patient. What is the loading dose, given the following: Vd = 0.5 L/kg, Cl = 0.04 L/kg/hr, t(1/2) −9.3 hr?

a) 0.5 L/kg * 60 kg * 7.5 mg/L = 225 mg/h, infusion
b) 0.5 L/kg * 60 kg * 7.5 mg/L = 225 mg, bolus
c) 0.04 L/kg/hr * 60 kg * 7.5 mg/L = 18 mg/h, infusion
d) 0.04 L/kg/hr * 60 kg * 7.5 mg/L = 18 mg, bolus

12. A target concentration of 7.5 mg/L of theophylline is required for a 60 kg patient.What is the steady state maintenance dose, given the following: Vd = 0.5 L/kg, Cl = 0.04 L/kg/hr, t(1/2) = 9.3 hr?
a) 0.5 L/kg * 60 kg * 7.5 mg/L = 225 mg/h, infusion
b) 0.5 L/kg * 60 kg * 7.5 mg/L = 225 mg, bolus
c) 0.04 L/kg/hr * 60 kg * 7.5 mg/L = 18 mg/h, infusion
d) 0.04 L/kg/hr * 60 kg * 7.5 mg/L = 18 mg, bolus

Answer Key

1-A 2-C 3-C 4-B 5-D 6-B 7-C 8-D 9-C 10-D 11-B 12-C

1.8 Drug Evaluation and Regulation

1. Which of the following is NOT an approach to drug development?
a) Chemical modification of a known molecule
b) Random screening for biologic activity (e.g. natural products)
c) Rational drug design
d) Combination of known drugs (e.g. Tylenol with codeine)

2. Drug screening for an anti-infectious agent would study the drug against a variety of infectious organisms (_____) and against non-infectious assays (_____).
a) Power; Specificity
b) Sensitivity; Side-effects
c) Activity; Selectivity
d) Selectivity; Activity

3.Subacute toxicity testing involves multiple doses over what time frame?
a) 1 week
b) 1 month
c) 6 months
d) 1 year

4. For the human clinical trials, what initial doses are used?
a) 1 – 2 NED
b) 1/2 – 1 NED
c) 1/10 – 1 NED
d) 1/100 – 1/10 NED

5. What is the minimal number of species tested (pregnant females) at selected organogenesis periods for teratogenesis? (e.g. Thalidomide, ethanol, Accutane, warfarin)
a) 1
b) 2
c) 3
d) 4

6. In the mutagenesis dominant lethal test, which of the following would be exposed to the test substance?
a) Pre-mating male
b) Pre-mating female
c) Post-mating male
d) Post-mating female (pregnant)

7. Which of the following teratogens is associated with absence of extremities?
a) Syphilis
b) Rubella
c) Thalidomide
d) Lithium

8. Which of the following is least likely to be involved in carcinogenesis?
a) Ethanol
b) Vinyl chloride
c) Urethane
d) Benzo[á]pyrene

9. What type of study for an Investigational New Drug (IND) involves neither the investigators or subjects knowing if the drug or placebo is being given?
a) Single-blind study
b) Double-blind study
c) Placebo
d) Positive-control

10. What type of study for an IND involves each subject receiving all treatment conditions?
a) Single-blind study
b) Double-blind study
c) Placebo (negative-control)
d) Crossover study

11. What type of study for an IND involves comparison with a placebo and anotherpreviously tested drug?
a) Single-blind study
b) Double-blind study
c) Placebo (negative-control)
d) Positive-control

12.What clinical trial phase involves many patients and often a double-blind study with the purpose to further explore the beneficial action of the drug and toxicities?
a) Phase 1
b) Phase 2
c) Phase 3
d) Phase 4

13. What clinical trial phase involves single- or double-blind studies under very controlled conditions with the purpose to determine therapeutic effect at tolerated doses?
a) Phase 1
b) Phase 2
c) Phase 3
d) Phase 4

14. What clinical trial phase involves submitting a New Drug Application (NDA), monitoring, and reporting by clinicians using the drug?
a) Phase 1
b) Phase 2
c) Phase 3
d) Phase 4

15. What clinical trial phase involves small does up to profound physiologic responses, or up to minor toxicity (pharmacokinetics)?
a) Phase 1
b) Phase 2
c) Phase 3
d) Phase 4

16. The Orphan Drug Amendment (1983) gives incentives for the development of orphan drugs, which treat diseases that affect less than how many patients?
a) 2,000
b) 20,000
c) 200,000
d) 2,000,000

17.Which of the following would NOT be a critique of the Prescription Drug User Fee Act (PDUFA, 1992)?
a) Obligates FDA to satisfy drug industry
b) Reduces FDA independence
c) Reduces FDA critical evaluation
d) Reduces drug approval process time

18. Which of the following drug safety categories for pregnancy is the highest risk, where studies have shown a significant risk to women and to the fetus?
a) A
b) B
c) C
d) X

Answer Key

01-D 02-D 03-C 04-D 05-B 06-A 07-C 08-A 09-B 10-D 11-D 12-C 13-B 14-D 15-A 16-C 17-D 18-D

1.9 Pharmacodynamics: Receptor Theory and Dose Response

1. Which of the following occurs on the extracellular domain of the lipid bilayer and not the cytoplasmic domain, with regard to drug action?
a) Ligand binding
b) Coupling with membrane associated molecules
c) Trafficking
d) Signaling

2. Which of the following drug targets involves inhibitors, false substrates, and a pro-drug type?
a) Receptors
b) Ion channels
c) Enzymes
d) Carriers

3. What is the correct order of bond strength, from strongest to weakest?
a) Van der Waals > Hydrogen > Ionic > Covalent
b) Ionic > Covalent > Hydrogen > Van der Waals
c) Covalent > Hydrogen > Ionic > Van der Waals
d) Covalent > Ionic > Hydrogen > Van der Waals

4. On a graded dose-response curve (or drug-receptor curve in a laboratory), at what point does response increase the most rapidly?
a) Initially
b) At EC50
c) At LD50
d) At 90% maximal response efficacy (Emax)

5. Which of the following is the equilibrium dissociation constant, where the concentration of free drug is at half-maximal binding?
a) EC50
b) Emax
c) Kd
d) Bmax

6. What kind of graph scaling is often used to compare EC50 to Kd?
a) Linear
b) Exponential
c) Semilog
d) Inverse

7. Which of the following drugs would require the most care when administrating, if the upper portion of the dose-response curve signified severe toxicity?
a) A
b) B
c) C
d) D

8. Which drug is the least efficacious?
a) A
b) B
c) C
d) D

9.Intrinsic activity is a drug's ability to elicit:
a) Strong receptor binding
b) Weak receptor binding
c) Response
d) Excretion

10. Which direction would a partial agonist shift the dose-response curve when compared to a full agonist?
a) To the left
b) To the right
c) Down
d) Up

11. Which direction would a competitive antagonist (plus agonist) shift the dose- response curve when compared to a full agonist?
a) To the left
b) To the right
c) Down
d) Up

12. Which direction would a non-competitive antagonist (plus agonist) shift the dose- response curve when compared to a full agonist?

a) To the left
b) To the right
c) Down
d) Down and possibly to the right

13. A competitive antagonist affects the agonist _____ and a non-competitive antagonist affect the agonist _____.
a) Potency; Efficacy
b) Efficacy; Potency
c) Duration; Speed
d) Speed; Duration

14. In which of the following cases could a dose-response curve be constructed?
a) Prevention of convulsions
b) Prevention of arrhythmias
c) Reduction of death
d) Reduction of fever

15. For most drugs, a frequency distribution of the response plotted against the log of the dose (quantal) produces what kind of curve?
a) Linear
b) Exponential
c) Logarithmic
d) Gaussian (normal) distribution

16. Generally, which of the following is the correct order as dosage is increased?
a) ED50 < LD50 < TD50
b) ED50 < TD50 < LD50
c) LD50 < TD50 < ED50
d) LD50 < ED50 < TD50

17. Which of the following is the median effective dose, or the dose at which 50% of the individuals exhibit the specified quantal response?
a) LD50
b) ED50
c) EC50
d) TD50

18.Which of the following is considered the therapeutic index (or ratio)?
a) T.I. = TD50 / ED50
b) T.I. = LD50 / ED50
c) T.I. = ED50 / TD50
d) A & B

19.Which of the following can be used as a relative indicator of the margin of safety of a drug?
a) LD50
b) ED50
c) EC50
d) T.I.

20.Which of the following is the most relevant use of therapeutic index?
a) Guide for toxicity in therapeutic the setting
b) Multiple measures of effectiveness are possible (e.g. aspirin)
c) Measure of impunity with which an overdose may be tolerated
d) Toxicities may be idiosyncratic (e.g. propranolol in asthmatics)

21. Which of the following refers to an increased intensity of response to a drug?
a) Idiosyncratic
b) Hyporeactive
c) Hyperreactive
d) Hypersensitive

22. Tachyphylaxis refers to which of the following?
a) Responsiveness increased rapidly after administration of a drug
b) Responsiveness decreased rapidly after administration of a drug
c) Responsiveness increased rapidly after maintenance of a drug (hypersensitive)
d) Responsiveness decreased rapidly after maintenance of a drug (desensitized)

Answer Key

01-A 02-C 03-D 04-C 05-C 06-C 07-D 08-B 09-C 10-C 11-B 12-D 13-A 14-D 15-D 16-B 17-B 18-D 19-D 20-C 21-C 22-B

1.10 Receptor-Effector Coupling

1. Which of the following would occur with an antagonist binding to a receptor and not an agonist?
a) Ion channel closed
b) Enzyme inhibited
c) Endogenous mediator blocked
d) Ion channel modulated

2. Nicotinic ACh receptors (ligand-gated) involve the movement of what ion across the membrane?
a) K+
b) Ca++
c) Cl-
d) Na+

3. The nicotinic receptor requires one molecule of ACh to bind to each of the two ____ receptors in order to activate the receptor and open the channel.
a) á (alpha)
b) â (beta)
c) g (gamma)
d) ä (delta)

4.GABA A receptors (ligand-gated) involve the movement of what ion across the membrane?
a) K+
b) Ca++
c) Cl-
d) Na+

5. Which of the following is increased in intracellular concentration due to second messengers such as IP3?
a) K+
b) Ca++
c) Cl-
d) Na+

6. Regulated by cytokines and growth factors, the Janus-Kinase JAK-STAT pathway results in which of the following?
a) Ion channel closing
b) Enzyme inhibition
c) Endogenous mediator blocking
d) Gene transcription

7. Which of the following describes the pathway of nitric oxide (NO)?
a) Stimulates guanylyl cyclase, increase cGMP concentration, vasodilation
b) Stimulates guanylyl cyclase, decreases cGMP concentration, vasodilation
c) Stimulates guanylyl cyclase, increase cGMP concentration, vasoconstriction
d) Inhibits guanylyl cyclase, increase cGMP concentration, vasodilation

8. Which of the following signaling mechanisms can involve heat-shock protein (hsp90)?

a) Intracellular receptors for lipid soluble ligands

b) Transmembrane receptors

c) G-protein coupled receptors

d) Ligand-gated ion channels

9. All of the following interact with ligand-gated ion channels EXCEPT:

a) Benzodiazepines

b) Insulin

c) Glutamate

d) Aspartate

10. Which of the following is NOT a second messenger associated with G proteins?

a) DAG

b) GDP

c) IP3

d) cAMP

11. Muscarinic ACh receptors and adrenergic receptors are associated with which of the following?

a) Intracellular receptors for lipid soluble ligands

b) Transmembrane receptors with enzymatic cytosolic domains

c) G-protein coupled receptors

d) Ligand-gated ion channels

12. In smooth muscle and glandular tissue, ACh binds to what muscarinic receptor, leading to the DAG cascade?

a) M1

b) M2

c) M3

d) M4

13. In the heart and intestines, what muscarinic receptor inhibits adenylyl cyclase activity?

a) M1

b) M2

c) M3

d) M4

14. Adrenergic á2 receptors ____ adenylyl cyclase and â receptors ____ adenylyl cyclase.
a) Stimulate; Stimulate
b) Stimulate; Inhibit
c) Inhibit; Inhibit
d) Inhibit; Stimulate

15. Which of the following is NOT a ligand-regulated transmembrane enzyme (agent)?
a) Insulin
b) EGP
c) PDFG
d) NO

16. Which of the following cytokine receptors (transmembrane enzyme) is antagonized by anakinra (Kineret), for treatment of rheumatoid arthritis?
a) Growth hormone
b) Erythropoietin
c) Interferons
d) Interleukin-1

17. Which of the following is NOT an intracellular receptor for lipid-soluble agent,which stimulates gene transcription in the nucleus by binding to DNA sequences?
a) Steroids
b) Vitamin A
c) Vitamin D
d) Thyroid

Answer Key

01-C 02-D 03-A 04-C 05-B 06-D 07-A 08-A 09-B 10-B 11-C 12-C 13-B 14-D 15-D 16-D 17-D

1.11 Autonomic Pharmacology: Sympathetic Nervous System

1. The sympathetic nervous system (SNS) and parasympathetic nervous system are divisions of which of the following?
a) Somatic nervous system division of peripheral nervous system
b) Somatic nervous system division of central nervous system
c) Autonomic nervous system division of peripheral nervous system
d) Autonomic nervous system division of central nervous system

2. Preganglionic sympathetic and parasympathetic fibers release ____, post-ganglionic parasympathetic fibers release ____ (for muscarinic cholinergic receptors), and postganglionic sympathetic fibers release ____ (for adrenergic receptors).

a) ACh; ACh; NE

b) ACh; NE; ACh

c) NE; ACh; NE

d) NE; NE; ACh

3.Which of the following adrenergic receptors is most commonly found pre-synaptic?

a) alpha 1

b) alpha 2

c) beta 1

d) beta 2

4. Which of the following describes the result of adrenal medulla stimulation?

a) Mass parasympathetic discharge, 85:15 ratio of epi:norepi

b) Mass parasympathetic discharge, 15:85 ratio of epi:norepi

c) Mass sympathetic discharge, 85:15 ratio of epi:norepi

d) Mass sympathetic discharge, 15:85 ratio of epi:norepi

5. Which of the following is transported into vesicles via the vesicular monoa-mine transporter (VMAT), uptake 2, a proton antiporter?

a) Epinephrine

b) Norepinephrine

c) Dopamine

6. Which of the following is co-stored and co-released with ATP?

a) Epinephrine

b) Norepinephrine

c) Dopamine

7. Which of the following form varicosities or en passant synapses, with the arrival of an action potential leading to Ca++ influx and exocytosis?

a) Presynaptic sympathetic

b) Presynaptic parasympathetic

c) Postsynaptic sympathetic

d) Postsynaptic parasympathetic

8. Which of the following methods of terminating axon response is NOT a target for drug action?
a) Reuptake via NE transporter (NET): Uptake 1
b) Metabolism of NE of inactive metabolite
c) NE diffusion away from synaptic cleft

9. NET is a symporter of what ion?
a) K+
b) Ca++
c) Cl-
d) Na+

10.Which of the following is recycled via VMAT into vesicles after response termination?
a) NE
b) L-DOPA
c) NET
d) EPI

11. Where is the cytosolic catecholamine metabolizing enzyme catechol-O-methyl transferase (COMT) primarily found?
a) Liver
b) GI tract
c) Placenta
d) Blood platelets

12.Which of the following receptor subtypes relaxes smooth muscle and causes liver glycogenolysis and gluconeogenesis?
a) alpha 1 (Gq/Gi/Go)
b) alpha 2 (Gi/Go)
c) beta 1 (Gs)
d) beta 2 (Gs)

13. Which of the following receptor subtypes causes vascular smooth muscle contraction and genitourinary smooth muscle contraction?
a) alpha 1 (Gq/Gi/Go)
b) alpha 2 (Gi/Go)
c) beta 1 (Gs)
d) beta 2 (Gs)

14. Which of the following receptor subtypes increases cardiac chronotropy (rate) and inotropy (contractility), increases AV-node conduction velocity, and increases rennin secretion in renal juxtaglomerular cells?
a) alpha 1 (Gq/Gi/Go)

b) alpha 2 (Gi/Go)

c) beta 1 (Gs)

d) beta 2 (Gs)

15. Which of the following receptor subtypes decreases insulin secretion from pancreatic beta-cells, decreases nerve cell norepinephrine release, and contracts vascular smooth muscle?

a) alpha 1 (Gq/Gi/Go)

b) alpha 2 (Gi/Go)

c) beta 1 (Gs)

d) beta 2 (Gs)

16. What type(s) of second messenger(s) interact with adenylyl cyclase?

a) alpha1

b) alpha2

c) beta

d) beta & alpha2

17. What type(s) of second messenger(s) are associated with phospholipase C (PLC)?

a) alpha1

b) beta 2

c) beta

d) beta & alpha 1

18. Which of the following adrenergic receptor activation mechanisms is involved with ephedrine, amphetamine, and tyramine?

a) Direct binding to the receptor

b) Promoting release of norepinephrine

c) Inhibiting reuptake of norepinephrine

d) Inhibiting inactivation of norepinephrine

19. Which of the following adrenergic receptor activation mechanisms is involved with MAO inhibitors?

a) Direct binding to the receptor

b) Promoting release of norepinephrine

c) Inhibiting reuptake of norepinephrine

d) Inhibiting inactivation of norepinephrine

20. Which of the following adrenergic receptor activation mechanisms is involved with tricyclic antidepressants and cocaine?

a) Direct binding to the receptor

b) Promoting release of norepinephrine
c) Inhibiting reuptake of norepinephrine
d) Inhibiting inactivation of norepinephrine

21. Which of the following is NOT true of catecholamines?
a) Non-polar
b) Cannot cross the blood-brain barrier
c) Cannot be used as an oral drug
d) Have brief duration

22. Which of the following is a long-acting (oral) alpha 1-agonist and not a short-acting (nasal spray, ophthalmic drops) alpha 1-agonist?
a) Phenylephrine
b) Oxymetazoline
c) Tetrahydrazaline
d) Pseudoephedrine

23. Which of the following would NOT be used as a topical vasoconstrictor for a patient with epistaxis (nasal pack soaked in drug)?
a) Phenylephrine
b) Epinephrine
c) Oymetazoline
d) Isoproterenol

24. alpha 1 drugs can be given with local anesthetics to vasoconstrictor and decrease blood flow to the side of administration. Which of the following should not be given above the web space?
a) Phenylephrine
b) Epinephrine
c) Methoxamine
d) Isoproterenol

25. Which of the following is the alpha 1 drug of choice (DOC) for retinal exams and surgery, giving mydiasis (dilation of iris)?
a) Ephedrine
b) Epinepherine
c) Oymetazoline
d) Phenylephrine

26. alpha 2-agonists are only approved for hypertension and work by decreasing sympathetic tone and increasing vagal tone. Which of the following is NOT a alpha 2-agonist?

a) Clonidine
b) Methyldopa
c) Guanabenz
d) Epinephrine

27. At the adrenergic synapse, what does alpha 2 do?
a) Stimulates NE release
b) Inhibits NE release
c) Stimulates ACh release
d) Inhibits ACh release

28. Which of the following agonists would be used for asthma patients or to delay premature labor?
a) alpha2-agonist
b) alpha1-agonist
c) beta 3-agonist
d) beta 2-agonist

29. Which of the following agonists would be used for cardiogenic shock, cardiac arrest, heart block, or heart failure?
a) alpha1-agonist
b) alpha2-agonist
c) beta 1-agonist
d) beta 2-agonist

30. Which of the following is NOT a beta 2-agonist?
a) Terbutaline
b) Ritodrine
c) Metaproterenol
d) Phenylepherine

31. beta 2 stimulation leads to an increase in the cellular uptake of what ion, and thus a decrease in plasma concentration of that ion?
a) K^+
b) Ca^{++}
c) Cl^-
d) Na^+

32. Dopamine receptor activation (D1) dilates renal blood vessels at low dose. At higher doses (treatment for shock), which of the following receptor is activated?
a) alpha 1

b) alpha 2
c) beta 1
d) beta 2

33. Which of the following responses to sympathetic stimulation would prevent receptors from being couples with G-proteins?
a) Sequestration
b) Down-regulation
c) Phosphorylation
d) none

34. Which of the following is the action of the indirect-acting sympathomimetic drug cocaine?
a) Stimulator of NET (uptake 1)
b) Inhibitor of NET (uptake 1)
c) Stimulator of VMAT (uptake 2)
d) Inhibitor of VMAT (uptake 2)

35. Tricyclic antidepressants (TCAs) have a great deal of side effects. Which of the following is the action of TCAs?
a) Stimulator of NET (uptake 1)
b) Inhibitor of NET (uptake 1)
c) Stimulator of VMAT (uptake 2)
d) Inhibitor of VMAT (uptake 2)

36. Which of the following is NOT a mixed sympathomimetic?
a) Amphetamine
b) Methamphetamine
c) Ephedrine
d) Phenylepherine

37. Prior to an operation to remove a pheochromocytoma (neuroendocrine tumor of the medulla of the adrenal glands), which of the following should be given to the patient?
a) alpha-agonist
b) alpha -blocker
c) beta -agonist
d) beta -blocker

38. Which of the following is NOT an indication for beta -blocker therapy?
a) Hypotension
b) Angina pectoris

c) Arrhythmias

d) Myocardial infarction

39. Which of the following beta -blockers is used for decreasing aqueous humor secretions from the ciliary body?

a) Propranolol

b) Nadolol

c) Carvedilol

d) Timolol

40. Which of the following is NOT considered cardioselective?

a) Metoprolol

b) Atenolol

c) Esmolol

d) Carvedilol

41. Blocking alpha2 presynaptic receptors will do which of the following?

a) Stimulate NE release

b) Inhibit NE release

c) Stimulate DA release

d) Inhibit DA release

42. Which of the following drugs irreversibly damages VMAT?

a) Tyramine

b) Guanethidine

c) Reserpine

d) Propranolol

43. Which of the following is the most likely to occur with parenteral administration of a alpha 1-agonist drug?

a) Hypotension

b) Hypertension

c) Tissue necrosis

d) Vasodilation

44. Which of the following agonists can have dose-related withdrawal syndrome if the drug is withdrawn too quickly, leading to rebound hypertension?

a) alpha1-agonist

b) alpha2-agonist

c) beta 1-agonist

d) beta 2-agonist

45. Which of the following agonists can have sedation and xerostomia (dry mouth) in 50% of patients starting therapy, sexual dysfunction in males, nauseas, dizziness, and sleep disturbances?
a) alpha1-agonist
b) alpha2-agonist
c) beta 1-agonist
d) beta 2-agonist

46. Which of the following agonists can cause hyperglycemia in diabetics?
a) alpha2-agonist
b) alpha1-agonist
c) beta 3-agonist
d) beta 2-agonist

47. Angina pectoris, tachycardia, and arrhythmias are possible adverse effects of which of the following agonists?
a) alpha2-agonist
b) alpha 1-agonist
c) beta 3-agonist
d) beta 1-agonist

48. If a patient is taking MAO inhibitors and ingests tyramine (red wine, aged cheese), which of the following acute responses is most likely? (sympathomimetic)
a) Stimulation of NE release
b) Inhibition of NE release
c) Stimulation of ACh release
d) Inhibition of ACh release

49.Which of the following occurs acutely, leading to a false neurotransmitter, with increased guanethidine? (sympathomimetic)
a) Stimulation of NE release
b) Inhibition of NE release
c) Stimulation of ACh release
d) Inhibition of ACh release

50. Major adverse affects of the alpha 1 blockade include reflex tachycardia and which of the following?
a) Orthostatic tachycardia
b) Orthostatic bradycardia
c) Orthostatic hypertension
d) Orthostatic hypotension

51. Which of the following effects would be intensified with the alpha 2 blockade?
a) Reflex tachycardia
b) Reflex bradycardia
c) Orthostatic hypertension
d) Orthostatic hypotension
e) Platelet clotting

52. Which of the following is NOT an adverse affect of the beta1 blockade?
a) Bradycardia
b) Decreased cardiac output
c) AV node block
d) Increased arrhythmias

53. Which of the following is the most severe adverse effect that has been associated with sudden termination of beta1-blockers?
a) Atrial fibrillation
b) Reflex bradycardia
c) Syncope (fainting)
d) Sudden death

54. Which of the following groups of patients is most at risk for adverse effect seen in beta 2-blockers?
a) Asthmatics
b) Congestive heart failure patients
c) Trauma patients
d) Diabetics

55. Which of the following can be detrimental in diabetics and also can lead to masking of tachycardia, which is indicative of hypoglycemia?
a) alpha1-blocker
b) alpha 2-blocker
c) beta 1-blocker
d) beta 2-blocker

Answer Key

01-C 02-A 03-B 04-C 05-C 06-B 07-C 08-C 09-D 10-A 11-A 12-D 13-A 14-C 15-B 16-D 17-A 18-B 19-D 20-C 21-A 22-D 23-D 24-B 25-D 26-E 27-B 28-D 29-C 30-D 31-A 32-C 33-C 34-B 35-B 36-B 37-B 38-A 39-C 40-D 41-A 42-C 43-B 44-B 45-B 46-D 47-D 48-A 49-A 50-D 51-A 52-D 53-D 54-A 55-D

1.12 Autonomic Pharmacology: Parasympathetic Nervous System

1.Which of the following is NOT true regarding the parasympathetic nervous system?
a) Is considered cranio-sacral
b) Involves rest and digestion functions
c) Has nicotinic receptors on cell bodies of all postganglionic neurons
d) Innervation of vascular smooth muscle

2. Where is acetyl CoA synthesized (pre-synthesis for ACh)?
a) Synaptic cleft
b) Cytosol
c) Mitochondria
d) Extracellular matrix

3. Which of the following locations contains choline from phosphatidylcho-line?
a) Milk
b) Liver
c) Eggs
d) Blood plasma

4. What part of the cholinergic synapse is affected by botulinum toxin?
a) ACh increased
b) ACh decreased
c) Muscarinic ACh receptor modified
d) Nicotinic ACh receptor modified

5. ACh is packaged into vesicles via what ACh ion antiporter?
a) K+
b) Ca++
c) Cl-
d) H+

6. Influx of what ion causes ACh release into the synaptic cleft, prior to ACh being terminated by acetylcholinesterase (AChE)?
a) K+
b) Ca++
c) Cl-
d) Na+

7. Nicotinic N2 receptors are the _____ subtype and nicotinic N1 receptors are the _____ subtype.

a) Neuronal; Muscular
b) Muscular; Neuronal
c) Nodal; Neuronal
d) Neuronal; Nodal

8. Which of the following best description of the drug nicotine?
a) Muscular subtype nicotinic agonist
b) Muscular subtype nicotinic antagonist
c) Neuronal subtype nicotinic agonist
d) Neuronal subtype nicotinic antagonist

9. Amanita muscaria (fly Amanita) is a fungal muscarinic agonist, which is most often associated with which side effect?
a) Tachycardia
b) Bradycardia
c) Euphoria
d) Hallucinations

10. Which of the following G-protein is associated with smooth muscle and glandular tissue, muscarinic receptor M3, mobilizing internal Ca++ and the DAG cascade?
a) Gs
b) Gi
c) Gq
d) Go

11. Which of the following G-protein is associated with heart and intestines, muscarinic receptor M2, decreasing adenylyl cyclase activity.
a) Gs
b) Gi
c) Gq
d) Go

12. The drugs bethanechol and pilocarpine are:
a) Acetylcholine agonists
b) Acetylcholine antagonists
c) Muscarinic agonists
d) Muscarinic antagonists

13. Which of the following is NOT a primary effect of stimulating muscarinic M receptors?

a) Release of nitric oxide (vasodilation)

b) Iris contraction (miosis)

c) Ciliary muscle contraction and accommodation of the lens (near vision)

d) Bronchi dilation and decreased bronchiole secretions

e) Salivary/lacrimal thin and watery secretions

14. Which of the following is NOT a primary effect of stimulating muscarinic M receptors?

a) Tachycardia, increased conduction velocity

b) Increased GI tract tone and secretions

c) Diaphoresis from sweat glands

d) Penile erection

15. What is bethanechol most commonly used for?

a) For decreasing heart rate

b) To decrease blood pressure (vasodilation)

c) For urinary retention

d) Decreasing intraocular pressure

16. What is pilocarpine most commonly used for?

a) For decreasing heart rate

b) To decrease blood pressure (vasodilation)

c) For urinary retention

d) Decreasing intraocular pressure

17. Which of the following is NOT a result of excessive cholinergic stimulation, as would be seen with a nerve agent or organophosphate poisoning?

a) Diarrhea

b) Diaphoresis

c) Mydriasis

d) Nausea

18.What type of drugs are atropine, scopolamine, and pirenzepine?

a) Acetylcholine agonists

b) Acetylcholine antagonists

c) Muscarinic agonists

d) Muscarinic antagonists

19. What drug is a natural alkaloid found in Solanaceae plants (deadly night-shade)?
a) Bethanechol
b) Pilocarpine
c) Pirenzepine
d) Atropine

20. What two clinical results of atropine facilitate opthalmoscopic examination?
a) Mydriasis (iris dilation) and increased lacrimation
b) Cycloplegia (ciliary paralysis) and miosis (iris constriction)
c) Miosis and increased lacrimation
d) Mydriasis and cycloplegia

21. Which of the following is an adverse affect of atropine?
a) Increased salivation
b) Blurred vision
c) Bradycardia
d) Diaphoresis

22. Which of the following is NOT a major symptom of atropine toxicity?
a) Blind as a bat
b) Red as a beet
c) Mad as a hatter
d) Wet as a towel

23. Which of the following topical ophthalmic drugs is also used for motion sickness? (injection, oral, or transdermal patch)
a) Atropine
b) Scopolamine
c) Homatropine
d) Tropicamide

24.Of the following mydriatics/cycloplegics, _____ last 7-10 days (longest) and _____ last 6 hours (shortest).
a) Atropine; Scopolamine
b) Scopolamine; Homatropine
c) Homatropine; Tropicamide
d) Atropine; Tropicamide

25. Butyrylcholinesterase (BuChE) is a nonspecific pseudocholinesterase located in glia, plasma, liver, and other organs. What type of local anesthetics are metabolized by BuChE(e.g. procaine), along with succinylcholine (paralytic)?
a) Ester
b) Ether
c) Amine
d) Alkane

26. Which of the following reversible cholinesterase inhibitors is used for atropine intoxication?
a) Neostigmine
b) Physostigmine
c) Endrophonium
d) Donepezil

27. Which of the following reversible cholinesterase inhibitors is used for anesthesia?
a) Neostigmine
b) Physostigmine
c) Endrophonium
d) Donepezil

28. Which of the following reversible cholinesterase inhibitors is used for Alzheimer disease?
a) Neostigmine
b) Physostigmine
c) Endrophonium
d) Donepezil

29. Which of the following cholinesterase inhibitors is NOT used for Myasthenia Gravis (MG)?
a) Neostigmine
b) Physostigmine
c) Endrophonium
d) Pyridostigmine

30. Which of the following is NOT an irreversible cholinesterase inhibitor (organophosphate AChE inhibitors)?
a) Tacrine
b) Echothiophate
c) Sarin, toban, soman
d) Malathion, parathion

31. By what mechanism do irreversible ACHE inhibitors permanently bind to the esteratic site enzyme?
a) Hydroxylation
b) Hydrolysis
c) Phosphorylation
d) Peptide

32. A MARK-1 autoinjection kit is given to certain medical and military personnel whomay be exposed to nerve agents or organophosphate pesticides. The kit has two drugs, anacetylcholinesterase inhibitor and a cholinesterase reactivator (antidote). What two drugswould you expect to be in this kit?
a) Pralidoxime (2-PAM) and echothiophate
b) Parathion and adenosine
c) Scopolamine and tropicamide
d) Atropine and pralidoxime (2-PAM)

33. Some organophosphate AChE inhibitor insecticides have a 40 hour half life. What is the approximate half life of soman?
a) 6 seconds
b) 6 minutes
c) 1 hour
d) 6 hours

34. What is currently the only ganglion blocker (shuts down entire ANS) still available in the United States?
a) Mecamylamine
b) Scopolamine
c) Echothiophate
d) Pralidoxime

35. Which of the following is NOT an effect of autonomic ganglion blocking?
a) Anhidrosis and xerostomia
b) Mydriasis
c) Tachycardia
d) Hypertension

Answer Key

01-D 02-C 03-D 04-B 05-D 06-B 07-A 08-C 09-D 10-C 11-B 12-C 13-D 14-A 15-C 16-D 17-C 18-D 19-D 20-D 21-B 22-D 23-B 24-D 25-A 26-B 27-A 28-D 29-B 30-A 31-C 32-D 33-B 34-A 35-D

2. Local anesthetics

1. Local anesthetics produce:
a) Analgesia, amnesia, loss of consciousness
b) Blocking pain sensation without loss of consciousness
c) Alleviation of anxiety and pain with an altered level of consciousness
d) A stupor or somnolent state

2. A good local anesthetic agent shouldn't cause:
a) Local irritation and tissue damage
b) Systemic toxicity
c) Fast onset and long duration of action
d) Vasodilatation

3. Most local anesthetic agents consist of:
a) Lipophylic group (frequently an aromatic ring)
b) Intermediate chain (commonly including an ester or amide)
c) Amino group
d) All of the above

4. Which one of the following groups is responsible for the duration of the local anesthetic action?
a) Intermediate chain
b) Lipophylic group
c) Ionizable group
d) All of the above

5. Indicate the local anesthetic agent, which has a shorter duration of action:
a) Lidocaine
b) Procaine
c) Bupivacaine
d) Ropivacaine

6. Which one of the following groups is responsible for the potency and the toxicity of local anesthetics?
a) Ionizable group
b) Intermediate chain
c) Lipophylic group
d) All of the above

7. Indicate the drug, which has greater potency of the local anesthetic action:
a) Lidocaine
b) Bupivacaine
c) Procaine
d) Mepivacaine

8. Ionizable group is responsible for:
a) The potency and the toxicity
b) The duration of action
c) The ability to diffuse to the site of action
d) All of the above

9. Which one of the following local anesthetics is an ester of benzoic acid?
a) Lidocaine
b) Procaine
c) Ropivacaine
d) Cocaine

10. Indicate the local anesthetic, which is an ester of paraaminobenzoic acid:
a) Mepivacaine
b) Cocaine
c) Procaine
d) Lidocaine

11. Which of the following local anesthetics is an acetanilide derivative?
a) Tetracaine
b) Lidocaine
c) Cocaine
d) Procaine

12. Indicate the local anesthetic, which is a toluidine derivative:
a) Lidocaine
b) Bupivacaine
c) Prilocaine
d) Procaine

13. Which of the following local anesthetics is a thiophene derivative?
a) Procaine
b) Ultracaine
c) Lidocaine
d) Mepivacaine

14. Local anesthetics are:
a) Weak bases
b) Weak acids
c) Salts
d) None of the above

15. For therapeutic application local anesthetics are usually made available as salts for the reasons of:
a) Less toxicity and higher potency
b) Higher stability and greater lipid solubility
c) Less local tissue damage and more potency
d) More stability and greater water solubility

16. Which of the following statements is not correct for local anesthetics?
a) In a tissue they exist either as an uncharged base or as a cation
b) A charged cationic form penetrates biologic membranes more readily than an uncharged form
c) Local anesthetics are much less effective in inflamed tissues
d) Low ph in inflamed tissues decreases the dissociation of nonionized molecules

17. Which one of the following statements about the metabolism of local anesthetics is incorrect?
a) Metabolism of local anesthetics occurs at the site of administration
b) Metabolism occurs in the plasma or liver but not at the site of administration
c) Ester group of anesthetics like procaine, are metabolized systemically by pseudocholinesterase
d) Amides such as lidocaine, are metabolized in the liver by microsomal mixed function oxidases

18. Indicate the anesthetic agent of choice in patient with a liver disease:
a) Lidocaine
b) Bupivacaine
c) Procaine
d) Etidocaine

19. Which of the following local anesthetics is preferable in patient with pseudocholinesterase deficiency?
a) Procaine
b) Ropivacaine
c) Tetracaine
d) Benzocaine

20. The primary mechanism of action of local anesthetics is:
a) Activation of ligand-gated potassium channels
b) Blockade of voltage-gated sodium channels
c) Stimulation of voltage-gated N-type calcium channels
d) Blockade the GABA-gated chloride channels

21. Which of the following local anesthetics is more water-soluble?
a) Tetracaine
b) Etidocaine
c) Procaine
d) Bupivacaine

22. Indicate the local anesthetic, which is more lipid-soluble:
a) Bupivacaine
b) Lidocaine
c) Mepivacaine
d) Procaine

23. The more lipophylic drugs:
a) Are more potent
b) Have longer duration of action
c) Bind more extensively to proteins
d) All of the above

24. Which of the following fibers is the first to be blocked?
a) Type A alpha fibers
b) B and C fibers
c) Type A beta fibers
d) Type A gamma fibers

25. Indicate the function, which the last to be blocked:
a) Pain, temperature
b) Muscle spindles
c) Motor function
d) Touch, pressure

26. Which of the following fibers participates in high-frequency pain transmission?
a) Type A delta and C fibers
b) Type A alpha fibers
c) Type B fibers
d) Type A beta fibers

27. Which of the following local anesthetics is an useful antiarrhythmic agent?
a) Cocaine
b) Lidocaine
c) Bupivacaine
d) Ropivacaine

28. Indicate the route of local anesthetic administration, which is associated with instillation within epidural or subarachnoid spaces:
a) Topical anesthesia
b) Infiltrative anesthesia
c) Regional anesthesia
d) Spinal anesthesia

29. The choice of a local anesthetic for specific procedures is usually based on:
a) The duration of action
b) Water solubility
c) Capability of rapid penetration through the skin or mucosa with limited tendency to diffuse away from the site of application
d) All of the above

30. Which of the following local anesthetics is a short-acting drug?
a) Procaine
b) Tetracaine
c) Bupivacaine
d) Ropivacaine

31. Indicate the local anesthetic, which is a long-acting agent:
a) Lidocaine
b) Bupivacaine
c) Procaine
d) Mepivacaine

32. The anesthetic effect of the agents of short and intermediate duration of action can not be prolonged by adding:
a) Epinephrine
b) Norepinephrine
c) Dopamine
d) Phenylephrine

33. A vasoconstrictor does not:
a) Retard the removal of drug from the injection site
b) Hence the chance of toxicity
c) Decrease the blood level
d) Reduce a local anesthetic uptake by the nerve

34. Vasoconstrictors are less effective in prolonging anesthetic properties of:
a) Procaine
b) Bupivacaine
c) Lidocaine
d) Mepivacaine

35. Which of the following local anesthetics is only used for surface or topical anesthesia?
a) Cocaine
b) Tetracaine
c) Procaine
d) Bupivacaine

36. Indicate the local anesthetic, which is mainly used for regional nerve block anesthesia:
a) Dibucaine
b) Bupivacaine
c) Tetracaine
d) Cocaine

37. Which of the following local anesthetics is used for infiltrative and regional anesthesia?
a) Procaine
b) Lidocaine
c) Mepivacaine
d) All of the above

38. Indicate the local anesthetic, which is used for spinal anesthesia:
a) Tetracaine
b) Cocaine
c) Dibucaine
d) Bupivacaine

39. Which of the following local anesthetics is called a universal anesthetic?
a) Procaine
b) Ropivacaine

c) Lidocaine
d) Bupivacaine

40. Most serious toxic reaction to local anesthetics is:
a) Seizures
b) Cardiovascular collapse
c) Respiratory failure
d) All of the above

41. Correct statements concerning cocaine include all of the following EXCEPT:
a) Cocaine is often used for nose and throat procedures
b) Limited use because of abuse potential
c) Myocardial depression and peripheral vasodilatation
d) Causes sympathetically mediated tachycardia and vasoconstriction

42. Which of the following local anesthetics is more cardiotoxic?
a) Procaine
b) Bupivacaine
c) Lidocaine
d) Mepivacaine

43. Most local anesthetics can cause:
a) Depression of abnormal cardiac pacemaker activity, excitability, conduction
b) Depression of the strength of cardiac contraction
c) Cardiovascular collapse
d) All of the above

44. Which one of the following local anesthetics causes methemoglobinemia?
a) Prilocaine
b) Procaine
c) Lidocaine
d) Ropivacaine

45. Procaine has all of the following properties EXCEPT:
a) It has ester linkage
b) Its metabolic product can inhibit the action of sulfonamides
c) It readily penetrates the skin and mucosa
d) It is relatively short-acting

46. Correct statements concerning lidocaine include all of the following EXCEPT:

a) It is an universal anesthetic

b) It has esteratic linkage

c) It widely used as an antiarrhythmic agent

d) It is metabolized in liver

47. Which of the following local anesthetics is more likely to cause allergic reactions?

a) Lidocaine

b) Bupivacaine

c) Procaine

d) Ropivacaine

48. Tetracaine has all of the following properties EXCEPT:

a) Slow onset

b) Low potency

c) Long duration

d) High toxicity

49. Correct statements concerning bupivacaine include all of the following EXCEPT:

a) It has low cardiotoxicity

b) It has amide linkage

c) It is a long-acting drug

d) An intravenous injection can lead to seizures

Answer Key

01-B 02-C 03-D 04-A 05-B 06-C 07-B 08-C 09-D 10-C 11-B 12-C 13-B 14-A 15-D 16-B 17-A 18-C 19-B 20-B 21-C 22-A 23-D 24-B 25-C 26-A 27-B 28-D 29-D 30-A 31-B 32-C 33-D 34-B 35-B 35-A 36-B 37-D 38-A 39-C 40-D 41-C 42-B 43-D 44-A 45-C 46-B 47-C 48-B 49-A

3. Cholinomimetic drugs

1. Acetylcholine is not a specific neurotransmitter at:

a) Sympathetic ganglia

b) Sympathetic postganglionic nerve endings

c) Parasympathetic ganglia

d) Parasympathetic postganglionic nerve endings

2. Muscarinic receptors are located in:

a) Autonomic ganglia

b) Skeletal muscle neuromuscular junctions

c) Autonomic effector cells

d) Sensory carotid sinus baroreceptor zone

3. Indicate the location of M_2 cholinoreceptor type:

a) Heart

b) Glands

c) Smooth muscle

d) Endothelium

4. The symptoms of mushroom poisoning include all of the following EXCEPT:

a) Salivation, lacrimation, nausea, vomiting

b) Dryness of mouth, hyperpyrexia, hallucination

c) Headache, abdominal colic

d) Bradycardia, hypotension and shock

5. Which of the following cholinomimetics activates both muscarinic and nicotinic receptors?

a) Lobeline

b) Pilocarpine

c) Nicotine

d) Bethanechol

6. Indicate a cholinomimetic agent, which is related to direct-acting drugs:

a) Edrophonium

b) Physostigmine

c) Carbachol

d) Isoflurophate

7. Characteristics of carbachol include all of the following EXCEPT:
a) It decreases intraocular pressure
b) It causes mydriasis
c) It exerts both nicotinic and muscarinic effects
d) It is resistant to acethylcholiesterase

8. Acetylcholine is not used in clinical practice because:
a) It is very toxic
b) The doses required are very high
c) It is very rapidly hydrolyzed
d) It is very costly

9. Parasympathomimetic drugs cause:
a) Bronchodilation
b) Mydriasis
c) Bradycardia
d) Constipation

10. Which of the following direct-acting cholinomimetics is mainly muscarinic in action?
a) Bethanechol
b) Carbachol
c) Acetylcholine
d) None of the above

11. Which of the following direct-acting cholinomimetics has the shortest duration of action?
a) Acetylcholine
b) Methacholine
c) Carbachol
d) Bethanechol

12. Bethanechol has all of the following properties EXCEPT:
a) It is extremely resistant to hydrolysis
b) Purely muscarinic in its action
c) It is used for abdominal urinary bladder distention
d) It exerts both nicotinic and muscarinic effects

13. A M-cholinimimetic agent is:
a) Carbachol
b) Pilocarpine
c) Acetylcholine
d) Bethanechol

14. Characteristics of pilocarpine include all of the following EXCEPT:
a) It is a tertiary amine alkaloid
b) It causes miosis and a decrease in intraocular pressure
c) Causes a decrease in secretory and motor activity of gut
d) It is useful in the treatment of glaucoma

15. Which of the following cholinomimetics is a plant derivative with lower potency than nicotine but with a similar spectrum of action?
a) Lobeline
b) Pilocarpine
c) Carbochol
d) Acetylcholine

16. Which of the following cholinomimetics is indirect-acting?
a) Lobeline
b) Edrophonium
c) Pilocarpine
d) Carbachol

17. The mechanism of action of indirect-acting cholinomimetic agents is:
a) Binding to and activation of muscarinic or nicotinic receptors
b) Inhibition of the hydrolysis of endogenous acetylcholine
c) Stimulation of the action of acetylcholinesterase
d) Releasing acetylcholine from storage sites

18. Indicate a reversible cholinesterase inhibitor:
a) Isoflurophate
b) Carbochol
c) Physostigmine
d) Parathion

19. Which of the following cholinesterase inhibitors is irreversible?
a) Physostigmine
b) Edrophonium
c) Neostigmine
d) Isoflurophate

20. Indicate cholinesterase activator:
a) Pralidoxime
b) Edrophonium
c) Pilocarpine
d) Isoflurophate

21. Isofluorophate increases all of the following effects except:
a) Lacrimation
b) Bronchodilation
c) Muscle twitching
d) Salivation

22. Indicate a cholinesterase inhibitor, which has an additional direct nicotinic agonist effect:
a) Edrophonium
b) Carbochol
c) Neostigmine
d) Lobeline

23. Cholinesterase inhibitors do not produce:
a) Bradycardia, no change or modest fall in blood pressure
b) Increased strength of muscle contraction, especially in muscles weakened by myasthenia gravis
c) Miosis and reduction of intraocular pressure
d) Dramatic hypertension and tachycardia

24. Which of the following cholinomimetics is commonly used in the treatment of glaucoma?
a) Pilocarpine
b) Lobeline
c) Acethylcholine
d) Neostigmine

25. Indicate the organophosphate cholinesterase inhibitor, which can be made up in an aqueous solution for ophthalmic use and retains its activity within a week:
a) Physoctigmine
b) Edrophonium
c) Echothiophate
d) Neostigmine

26. Which of the following cholinomimetics is most widely used for paralytic ileus and atony of the urinary bladder?
a) Lobeline
b) Neostigmine
c) Pilocarpine
d) Echothiophate

27. Chronic long-term therapy of myasthenia is usually accomplished with:
a) Edrophonium
b) Neostigmine
c) Echothiophate
d) Carbachol

28. Which of the following cholinomimetics is a drug of choice for reversing the effects of nondepolarizing neuromuscular relaxants?
a) Echothiophate
b) Physostigmine
c) Edrophonium
d) Pilocarpine

29. Indicate the reversible cholinesterase inhibitor, which penetrates the blood-brain barrier:
a) Physostigmine
b) Edrophonium
c) Neostigmine
d) Piridostigmine

30. Which of the following cholinomimetics is used in the treatment of atropine intoxication?
a) Neostigmine
b) Carbochol
c) Physostigmine
d) Lobeline

31. The symptoms of excessive stimulation of muscarinic receptors include all of the following EXCEPT:
a) Abdominal cramps, diarrhea
b) Increased salivation, excessive bronchial secretion
c) Miosis, bradycardia
d) Weakness of all skeletal muscles

32. The excessive stimulation of muscarinic receptors by pilocarpine and choline esters is blocked competitively by:
a) Edrophonium
b) Atropine
c) Pralidoxime
d) Echothiophate

33. The toxic effects of a large dose of nicotine include all of the following EXCEPT:

a) Hypotension and bradycardia

b) Convulsions, coma and respiratory arrest

c) Skeletal muscle depolarization blockade and respiratory paralysis

d) Hypertension and cardiac arrhythmias

34. The dominant initial sights of acute cholinesterase inhibitors intoxication include all of the following except:

a) Salivation, sweating

b) Mydriasis

c) Bronchial constriction

d) Vomiting and diarrhea

35. Which of the following drugs is used for acute toxic effects of organophosphate cholinesterase inhibitors?

a) Atropine

b) Pilocarpine

c) Pralidoxime

d) Edrophonium

Answer Key

01-B 02-C 03-A 04-D 05-D 06-C 07-B 08-C 09-C 10-A 11-A 12-D 13-B 14-C 15-A 16-B 17-B 18-C 19-D 20-A 21-B 22-C 23-D 24-A 25-C 26-B 27-B 28-C 29-A 30-C 31-D 32-B 33-A 34-B 35-C

4. Cholinoreceptor blocking drugs

1. The group of nicotinic receptor-blocking drugs consists of:
a) Ganglion-blockers
b) Atropine-similar drugs
c) Neuromuscular junction blockers
d) Both a and c

2. M₃receptor subtype is located:
a) In the myocardium
b) In sympathetic postganglionic neurons
c) On effector cell membranes of glandular and smooth muscle cells
d) On the motor end plates

3. Which of the following drugs is both a muscarinic and nicotinic blocker?
a) Atropine
b) Benztropine
c) Hexamethonium
d) Succinylcholine

4. Indicate a muscarinic receptor-blocking drug:
a) Scopolamine
b) Pipecuronium
c) Trimethaphan
d) Pilocarpine

5. Which of the following agents is a ganglion-blocking drug?
a) Homatropine
b) Hexamethonium
c) Rapacuronium
d) Edrophonium

6. Indicate the skeletal muscle relaxant, which is a depolarizing agent:
a) Vencuronium
b) Scopolamine
c) Succinylcholine
d) Hexamethonium

7. Which of the following drugs is a nondepolarizing muscle relaxant?
a) Pancuronium
b) Succinylcholine
c) Hexamethonium
d) Scopolamine

8. Indicate the drug, which is rapidly and fully distributed into CNS and has a greater effect than most other antimuscarinic agents?
a) Atropine
b) Scopolamine
c) Homatropine
d) Ipratropium

9. The effect of the drug on parasympathetic function declines rapidly in all organs EXCEPT:
a) Eye
b) Heart
c) Smooth muscle organs
d) Glands

10. The mechanism of atropine action is:
a) Competitive ganglion blockade
b) Competitive muscarinic blockade
c) Competitive neuromuscular blockade
d) Noncompetitive neuromuscular blockade

11. The tissues most sensitive to atropine are:
a) The salivary, bronchial and sweat glands
b) The gastric parietal cells
c) Smooth muscle and autonomic effectors
d) The heart

12. Atropine is highly selective for:
a) M_1 receptor subtype
b) M_2 receptor subtype
c) M_3 receptor subtype
d) All of the above

13. Which of the following antimuscarinic drugs is often effective in preventing or reversing vestibular disturbances, especially motion sickness?
a) Atropine
b) Ipratropium

c) Scopolamine
d) Homatropine

14. Atropine causes:
a) Miosis, a reduction in intraocular pressure and cyclospasm
b) Mydriasis, a rise in intraocular pressure and cycloplegia
c) Miosis, a rise in intraocular pressure and cycloplegia
d) Mydriasis, a rise in intraocular pressure and cyclospasm

15. Patients complain of dry or "sandy" eyes when receiving large doses of:
a) Atropine
b) Hexamethonium
c) Pilocarpine
d) Carbachol

16. All of the following parts of the heart are very sensitive to muscarinic receptor blockade except:
a) Atria
b) Sinoatrial node
c) Atrioventricular node
d) Ventricle

17. Atropine causes:
a) Bradycardia, hypotension and bronchoconstriction
b) Tachycardia, little effect on blood pressure and bronchodilation
c) Decrease in contractile strength, conduction velocity through the AV node
d) Tachycardia, hypertensive crisis and bronchodilation

18. Atropine is frequently used prior to administration of inhalant anesthetics to reduce:
a) Muscle tone
b) Secretions
c) Nausea and vomiting
d) All of the above

19. Atropine is now rarely used for the treatment of peptic ulcer because of:
a) Slow gastric empting and prolongation of the exposure of the ulcer bed to acid
b) Low efficiency and necessity of large doses
c) Adverse effects
d) All of the above

$_1$blocker?

20. Which of the following antimuscarinic drugs is a selective M

a) Atropine

b) Scopolamine

c) Pirenzepine

d) Homatropine

21. Atropine causes:

a) Spasmolitic activity

b) Intestinal hypermotility

c) Stimulation of contraction in the gut

d) Stimulation of secretory activity

22. Which of the following drugs is useful in the treatment of uterine spasms?

a) Carbachol

b) Vecuronium

c) Atropine

d) Edrophonium

23. Atropine may cause a rise in body temperature (atropine fever):

a) In adults

b) In pregnant women

c) In infants and children

d) All of the above

24. The pharmacologic actions of scopolamine most closely resemble those of:

a) Hexamethonium

b) Atropine

c) Succinylcholine

d) Pilocarpine

25. Compared with atropine, scopolamine has all of the following properties EXCEPT:

a) More marked central effect

b) Less potent in decreasing bronchial, salivary and sweat gland secretion

c) More potent in producing mydriasis and cycloplegia

d) Lower effects on the heart, bronchial muscle and intestines

26. Which of the following drugs is useful in the treatment of Parkinson's disease?

a) Benztropine

b) Edrophonium

c) Succinylcholine

d) Hexamethonium

27. Indicate the antimuscarinic drug, which is used as a mydriatic:
a) Pilocarpine
b) Neostigmine
c) Homatropine
d) Ipratropium

28. Which of the following agents is used as an inhalation drug in asthma?
a) Atropine
b) Ipratropium
c) Lobeline
d) Homatropine

29. Which of the following agents is most effective in regenerating cholinesterase associated with skeletal muscle neuromuscular junctions?
a) Suscinilcholine
b) Pralidoxime
c) Pirenzepine
d) Propiverine

30. Indicate an antimuscarinic drug, which is effective in the treatment of mushroom poising:
a) Pralidoxime
b) Pilocarpine
c) Homatropine
d) Atropine

31. Antimuscarinics are used in the treatment of the following disorders EXCEPT:
a) Motion sickness
b) Glaucoma
c) Hyperhidrosis
d) Asthma

32. The atropine poisoning includes all of the following symptoms EXCEPT:
a) Mydriasis, cycloplegia
b) Hyperthermia, dry mouth, hot and flushed skin
c) Agitation and delirium
d) Bradicardia, orthostatic hypotension

33. The treatment of the antimuscarinic effects can be carried out with:
a) Neostigmine

b) Hexametonium

c) Homatropine

d) Acetylcholine

34. Contraindications to the use of antimuscarinic drugs are all of the following except:
a) Glaucoma

b) Myasthenia

c) Bronchial asthma

d) Paralytic ileus and atony of the urinary bladder

35. Hexamethonium blocks the action of acethylcholine and similar agonists at:
a) Muscarinic receptor site

b) Neuromuscular junction

c) Autonomic ganglia

d) Axonal transmission

36. The applications of the ganglion blockers have disappeared because of all of the following reasons EXCEPT:
a) Orthostatic hypotension

b) Lack of selectivity

c) Homeostatic reflexes block

d) Respiratory depression

37. Which of the following agents is a short-acting ganglion blocker?
a) Homatropine

b) Trimethaphane

c) Hexamethonium

d) Pancuronium

38. Indicate the ganglion-blocking drug, which can be taken orally for the treatment of hypertension?
a) Mecamylamine

b) Scopolamine

c) Trimethaphane

d) Vecocuronium

39. The systemic effects of hexamethonium include all of the following EXCEPT:
a) Reduction of both peripheral vascular resistance and venous return
b) Partial mydriasis and loss of accommodation
c) Constipation and urinary retention
d) Stimulation of thermoregulatory sweating

40. Ganglion blocking drugs are used for the following emergencies EXCEPT:
a) Hypertensive crises
b) Controlled hypotension
c) Cardiovascular collapse
d) Pulmonary edema

41. Agents that produce neuromuscular blockade act by inhibiting:
a) Interaction of acetylcholine with cholinergic receptors
b) Release of acetylcholine from prejunctional membrane
c) Packaging of acetylcholine into synaptic vesicles
d) Reuptake of acetylcholine into the nerve ending

42. Skeletal muscle relaxation and paralysis can occur from interruption of functions at several sites, including all of the following EXCEPT:
a) Nicotinic acethylcholine receptors
b) Muscarinic acethylcholine receptors
c) The motor end plate
d) Contractile apparatus

43. Nondepolarisation neuromuscular blocking agents:
a) Block acetylcholine reuptake
b) Prevent access of the transmitter to its receptor and depolarization
c) Block transmission by an excess of a depolarizing agonist
d) All of the above

44. Which of the following drugs has "double-acetylcholine" structure?
a) Rocuronium
b) Carbachol
c) Atracurium
d) Succylcholine

45. Indicate the long-acting neuromuscular blocking agent:
a) Rapacuronium
b) Mivacurium
c) Tubocurarine
d) Rocuronium

46. Which of the following neuromuscular blocking drugs is an intermediate-duration muscle relaxant?

a) Vecuronium

b) Tubocurarine

c) Pancuronium

d) Rapacuronium

47. Indicate the nondepolarizing agent, which has the fastest onset of effect?

a) Succinylcholine

b) Rapacuronium

c) Pancuronium

d) Tubocurarine

48. Indicate the neuromuscular blocker, whose breakdown product readily crosses the blood-brain barrier and may cause seizures:

a) Pancuronium

b) Succinylcholine

c) Tubocurarine

d) Atracurium

49. Which competitive neuromuscular blocking agent could be used in patients with renal failure?

a) Atracurium

b) Succinylcholine

c) Pipecuronium

d) Doxacurium

50. Indicate the nondepolarizing agent, which has short duration of action:

a) Succinylcholine

b) Tubocurarine

c) Mivacurium

d) Pancuronium

51. Which depolarizing agent has the extremely brief duration of action?

a) Mivacurium

b) Rapacuronium

c) Rocuronium

d) Succinylcholine

52. Neuromuscular blockade by both succinylcholine and mivacurium may be prolonged in patients with:
a) Renal failure
b) An abnormal variant of plasma cholinesterase
c) Hepatic disease
d) Both b and c

53. Depolarizing agents include all of the following properties EXCEPT:
a) Interact with nicotinic receptor to compete with acetylcholine without receptor activation
b) React with the nicotinic receptor to open the channel and cause depolarisation of the end plate
c) Cause desensitization, noncompetive block manifested by flaccid paralysis
d) Cholinesterase inhibitors do not have the ability to reverse the blockade

54. Which of the following neuromuscular blockers causes transient muscle fasciculations?
a) Mivacurium
b) Pancuronium
c) Succinylcholine
d) Tubocurarine

55. Indicate muscles, which are more resistant to block and recover more rapidly:
a) Hand
b) Leg
c) Neck
d) Diaphragm

56. Which neuromuscular blocking agent has the potential to cause the greatest release of histamine?
a) Succylcholine
b) Tubocurarine
c) Pancuronium
d) Rocuronium

57. Which of the following muscular relaxants causes hypotension and bronchospasm?
a) Vecuronium
b) Succinylcholine
c) Tubocurarine
d) Rapacuronium

58. Indicate the neuromuscular blocker, which causes tachycardia:
a) Tubocurarine
b) Atracurium
c) Pancuronium
d) Succinylcholine

59. Which of the following neuromuscular blocking agents cause cardiac arrhythmias?
a) Vecuronium
b) Tubocurarine
c) Rapacuronium
d) Succinylcholine

60. Effects seen only with depolarizing blockade include all of the following EXCEPT:
a) Hypercaliemia
b) A decrease in intraocular pressure
c) Emesis
d) Muscle pain

61. Which neuromuscular blocking agent is contraindicated in patients with glaucoma?
a) Tubocurarine
b) Succinylcholine
c) Pancuronium
d) Gallamine

62. Indicate the following neuromuscular blocker, which would be contraindicated in patients with renal failure:
a) Pipecuronium
b) Succinylcholine
c) Atracurium
d) Rapacuronium

63. All of the following drugs increase the effects of depolarizing neuromuscular blocking agents EXCEPT:
a) Aminoglycosides
b) Antiarrhythmic drugs
c) Nondepolarizing blockers
d) Local anesthetics

64. Which of the following diseases can augment the neuromuscular blockade produced by nondepolarizing muscle relaxants?
a) Myasthenia gravis
b) Burns
c) Asthma
d) Parkinsonism

65. Indicate the agent, which effectively antagonizes the neuromuscular blockade caused by nondepolarizing drugs:
a) Atropine
b) Neostigmine
c) Acetylcholine
d) Pralidoxime

Answer Key

01-D 02-C 03-B 04-A 05-B 06-C 07-A 08-B 09-A 10-B 11-A 12-D 13-C 14-B 15-A 16-D 17-B 18-B 19-D 20-C 21-A 22-C 23-C 24-B 25-B 26-A 27-C 28-B 29-B 30-D 31-B 32-D 33-A 34-C 35-C 36-D 37-B 38-A 39-D 40-C 41-A 42-D 43-B 44-D 45-C 46-A 47-B 48-D 49-A 50-C 51-D 52-D 53-A 54-C 55-D 56-B 57-C 58-C 59-D 60-D 61-B 62-A 63-C 64-A 65-B

5. Adrenoreceptor activating drugs

1. Sympathetic stimulation is mediated by:
a) Release of norepinephrine from nerve terminals
b) Activation of adrenoreceptors on postsynaptic sites
c) Release of epinephrine from the adrenal medulla
d) All of the above

2. Characteristics of epinephrine include all of the following EXCEPT:
a) It is synthesized into the adrenal medulla
b) It is synthesized into the nerve ending
c) It is transported in the blood to target tissues
d) It directly interacts with and activates adrenoreceptors

3. Which of the following sympathomimetics acts indirectly?
a) Epinephrine
b) Norepinephrine
c) Ephedrine
d) Methoxamine

4. Indirect action includes all of the following properties EXCEPT:
a) Displacement of stored catecholamines from the adrenergic nerve ending
b) Inhibition of reuptake of catecholamines already released
c) Interaction with adrenoreceptors
d) Inhibition of the release of endogenous catecholamines from peripheral adrenergic neurons

5. Catecholamine includes following EXCEPT:
a) Ephedrine
b) Epinephrine
c) Isoprenaline
d) Norepinephrine

6. Epinephrine decreases intracellular camp levels by acting on:
a) α_1 receptor
b) α_2 receptor
c) beta$_1$ receptor
d) beta$_2$ receptor

7. Which of the following statements is not correct?
a) ALFA receptors increase arterial resistence, whereas $beta_2$receptor promote smooth muscle relaxation
b) The skin and splanchic vessels have predominantly alfa receptors
c) Vessels in a skeletal muscle may constrict or dilate depending on whether alfa or $beta_2$ receptors are activated
d) Skeletal muscle vessels have predominantly alfa receptors and constrict in the presence of epinephrine and norepinephrine

8. Direct effects on the heart are determined largely by:
a) $Alfa_1$receptor
b) $Alfa_2$receptor
c) $Beta_1$ receptor
d) $Beta_2$receptor

9. Which of the following effects is related to direct $beta_1$-adrenoreceptor stimulation?
a) Bronchodilation
b) Vasodilatation
c) Tachycardia
d) Bradycardia

10. Distribution of alfa adrenoreceptor subtypes is associated with all of the following tissues except those of:
a) Heart
b) Blood vessels
c) Prostate
d) Pupillary dilator muscle

11. Beta adrenoreceptor subtypes is contained in all of the following tissues EXCEPT:
a) Bronchial muscles
b) Heart
c) Pupillary dilator muscle
d) Fat cells

12. In which of the following tissues both alfa and $beta_1$adrenergic stimulation produces the same effect?
a) Blood vessels
b) Intestine
c) Uterus
d) Bronchial muscles

13. The effects of sympathomimetics on blood pressure are associated with their effects on:
a) The heart
b) The peripheral resistance
c) The venous return
d) All of the above

14. A relatively pure alfa agonist causes all of the following effects EXCEPT:
a) Increase peripheral arterial resistance
b) Increase venous return
c) Has no effect on blood vessels
d) Reflex bradycardia

15. A nonselective beta receptor agonist causes all of the following effects Except:
a) Increase cardiac output
b) Increase peripheral arterial resistance
c) Decrease peripheral arterial resistance
d) Decrease the mean pressure

16. Which of the following statement is not correct?
a) Alfa agonists cause miosis
b) Alfa agonists cause mydriasis
c) Beta antagonists decrease the production of aqueous humor
d) Alfa agonists increase the outflow of aqueous humor from the eye

17. A bronchial smooth muscle contains:
a) Alfa$_1$receptor
b) Alfa$_2$receptor
c) Beta $_1$receptor
d) Beta $_2$ receptor

18. All of the following agents are beta receptor agonists EXCEPT:
a) Epinephrine
b) Isoproterenol
c) Methoxamine
d) Dobutamine

19. Which of the following drugs causes bronchodilation without significant cardiac stimulation?
a) Isoprenaline
b) Terbutaline
c) Xylometazoline
d) Methoxamine

20. Alfa-receptor stimulation includes all of the following effects EXCEPT:
a) Relaxation of gastrointestinal smooth muscle
b) Contraction of bladder base, uterus and prostate
c) Stimulation of insulin secretion
d) Stimulation of platelet aggregation

21. Beta$_1$receptor stimulation includes all of the following effects EXCEPT:
a) Increase in contractility
b) Bronchodilation
c) Tachycardia
d) Increase in conduction velocity in the atrioventricular node

22. Beta$_2$receptor stimulation includes all of the following effects EXCEPT:
a) Stimulation of renin secretion
b) Fall of potassium concentration in plasma
c) Relaxation of bladder, uterus
d) Tachycardia

23. Hyperglycemia induced by epinephrine is due to:
a) Gluconeogenesis (beta$_2$)
b) Inhibition of insulin secretion (alfa)
c) Stimulation of glycogenolysis (beta$_2$)
d) All of the above

24. Which of the following effects is associated with beta$_3$-receptor stimulation?
a) Lipolysis
b) Decrease in platelet aggregation
c) Bronchodilation
d) Tachycardia

25. Which of the following statements is not correct?
a) Epinephrine acts on both alfa- and beta-receptors
b) Norepinephrine has a predominantly beta action
c) Methoxamine has a predominantly alfa action
d) Isoprenaline has a predominantly beta action

26. Indicate the drug, which is a direct-acting both alfa- and beta-receptor agonist:

a) Norepinephrine

b) Methoxamine

c) Isoproterenol

d) Ephedrine

27. Which of the following agents is an alfa$_1$alfa$_2$beta$_1$beta$_2$receptor agonist?

a) Methoxamine

b) Albuterol

c) Epinephrine

d) Norepinephrine

28. Indicate the direct-acting sympathomimetic, which is an alfa$_1$alfa$_2$beta$_1$ receptor agonist:

a) Isoproterenol

b) Ephedrine

c) Dobutamine

d) Norepinephrine

29. Which of the following agents is an alfa$_1$-selective agonist?

a) Norepinephrine

b) Methoxamine

c) Ritodrine

d) Ephedrine

30. Indicate the alfa$_2$-selective agonist:

a) Xylometazoline

b) Epinephrine

c) Dobutamine

d) Methoxamine

31. Which of the following agents is a nonselective beta receptor agonist?

a) Norepinephrine

b) Terbutaline

c) Isoproterenol

d) Dobutamine

32. Indicate the beta$_1$-selective agonist:

a) Isoproterenol

b) Dobutamine

c) Metaproterenol

d) Epinephrine

33. Which of the following sympathomimetics is a beta$_2$-selective agonist?
a) Terbutaline
b) Xylometazoline
c) Isoproterenol
d) Dobutamine

34. Indicate the indirect-acting sympathomimetic agent:
a) Epinephrine
b) Phenylephrine
c) Ephedrine
d) Isoproterenol

35. Epinephrine produces all of the following effects EXCEPT:
a) Positive inotropic and chronotropic actions on the heart (beta$_1$receptor)
b) Increase peripheral resistance (alfa receptor)
c) Predominance of alfa effects at low concentration
d) Skeletal muscle blood vessel dilatation (beta$_2$receptor)

36. Epinephrine produces all of the following effects EXCEPT:
a) Decrease in oxygen consumption
b) Bronchodilation
c) Hyperglycemia
d) Mydriasis

37. Epinephrine is used in the treatment of all of the following disorders EXCEPT:
a) Bronchospasm
b) Anaphylactic shock
c) Cardiac arrhythmias
d) Open-angle glaucoma

38. Compared with epinephrine, norepinephrine produces all of the following effects EXCEPT:
a) Similar effects on beta$_1$receptors in the heart and similar potency at an alfa receptor
b) Decrease the mean pressure below normal before returning to the control value
c) Significant tissue necrosis if injected subcutaneously
d) Increase both diastolic and systolic blood pressure

39. Norepinephrine produces:
a) Vasoconstriction
b) Vasodilatation
c) Bronchodilation
d) Decresed potassium concentration in the plasma

40. Which of the following direct-acting drugs is a relatively pure alfa agonist, an effective mydriatic and decongestant and can be used to raise blood pressure?
a) Epinephrine
b) Norepinephrine
c) Phenylephrine
d) Ephedrine

41. Characteristics of methoxamine include all of the following EXCEPT:
a) It is a direct-acting alfa$_1$-receptor agonist
b) It increases heart rate, contractility and cardiac output
c) It causes reflex bradycardia
d) It increases total peripheral resistance

42. Which of the following agents is an alfa$_2$-selective agonist with ability to promote constriction of the nasal mucosa?
a) Xylometazoline
b) Phenylephrine
c) Methoxamine
d) Epinephrine

43. Indicate the sympathomimetic, which may cause hypotension, presumably because of a clonidine-like effect:
a) Methoxamine
b) Phenylephrine
c) Xylometazoline
d) Isoproterenol

44. Isoproterenol is:
a) Both an alfa- and beta-receptor agonist
b) beta$_1$-selective agonist
c) beta$_2$-selective agonist
d) Nonselective beta receptor agonist

45. Isoproterenol produces all of the following effects EXCEPT:
a) Increase in cardiac output
b) Fall in diastolic and mean arterial pressure
c) Bronchoconstriction
d) Tachycardia

46. Characteristics of dobutamine include all of the following EXCEPT:
a) It is a relatively $beta_1$-selective synthetic catecholamine
b) It is used to treat bronchospasm
c) It increases atrioventricular conduction
d) It causes minimal changes in heart rate and systolic pressure

47. Characteristics of salmeterol include all of the following EXCEPT:
a) It is a potent selective $beta_2$ agonist
b) It causes uterine relaxation
c) It stimulates heart rate, contractility and cardiac output
d) It is used in the therapy of asthma

48. Characteristics of ephedrine include all of the following EXCEPT:
a) It acts primarily through the release of stored cathecholamines
b) It is a mild CNS stimulant
c) It causes tachyphylaxis with repeated administration
d) It decreases arterial pressure

49. Ephedrine causes:
a) Miosis
b) Bronchodilation
c) Hypotension
d) Bradycardia

50. Compared with epinephrine, ephedrine produces all of the following features EXCEPT:
a) It is a direct-acting sympathomimetic
b) It has oral activity
c) It is resistant to MAO and has much longer duration of action
d) Its effects are similar, but it is less potent

51. Which of the following sympathomimetics is preferable for the treatment of chronic orthostatic hypotension?
a) Epinephrine
b) Norepinephrine
c) Ephedrine
d) Salmeterol

52. Indicate the sympathomimetic drug, which is used in a hypotensive emergency:
a) Xylometazoline
b) Ephedrine
c) Terbutaline
d) Phenylephrine

53. Which of the following sympathomimetics is preferable for the emergency therapy of cardiogenic shock?
a) Epinephrine
b) Dobutamine
c) Isoproterenol
d) Methoxamine

54. Indicate the sympathomimetic agent, which is combined with a local anesthetic to prolong the duration of infiltration nerve block:
a) Epinephrine
b) Xylometazoline
c) Isoproterenol
d) Dobutamine

55. Which of the following sympathomimetics is related to short-acting topical decongestant agents?
a) Xylometazoline
b) Terbutaline
c) Phenylephrine
d) Norepinephrine

56. Indicate the long-acting topical decongestant agents:
a) Epinephrine
b) Norepinephrine
c) Phenylephrine
d) Xylometazoline

57. Which of the following topical decongestant agents is an alfa$_2$-selective agonist?
a) Phenylephrine
b) Xylometazoline
c) Ephedrine
d) Epinephrine

58. Indicate the sympathomimetic, which may be useful in the emergency management of cardiac arrest:
a) Methoxamine
b) Phenylephrine
c) Epinephrine
d) Xylometazoline

59. Which of the following sympathomimetics is used in the therapy of bronchial asthma?
a) Formoterol
b) Norepinephrine
c) Methoxamine
d) Dobutamine

60. Indicate the agent of choice in the emergency therapy of anaphylactic shock:
a) Methoxamine
b) Terbutaline
c) Norepinephrine
d) Epinephrine

61. Which of the following sympathomimetics is an effective mydriatic?
a) Salmeterol
b) Phenylephrine
c) Dobutamine
d) Norepinephrine

62. The adverse effects of sympathomimetics include all of the following EXCEPT:
a) Drug-induced parkinsonism
b) Cerebral hemorrhage or pulmonary edema
c) Myocardial infarction
d) Ventricular arrhythmias

Answer Key

01-D 02-B 03-C 04-C 05-A 06-B 07-D 08-C 09-C 10-A 11-C 12-B 13-D 14-C 15-B 16-A 17-D 18-C 19-B 20-C 21-B 22-D 23-D 24-A 25-B 26-A 27-C 28-D 29-B 30-B 31-C 32-B 33-A 34-C 35-C 36-A 37-C 38-B 39-A 40-C 41-B 42-A 43-C 44-D 45-C 46-B 47-C 48-D 49-B 50-A 51-C 52-D 53-B 54-A 55-C 56-D 57-B 58-C 59-A 60-D 61-B 62-A

6. Adrenoreceptor antagonist drugs

1. Which of the following drugs is a nonselective alfa receptor antagonist?
a) Prazosin
b) Phentolamine
c) Metoprolol
d) Reserpine

2. Indicate the alfa$_1$-selective antagonist:
a) Phentolamine
b) Dihydroergotamine
c) Prazosin
d) Labetalol

3. Which of the following agents is an alfa$_2$-selective antagonist?
a) Yohimbine
b) Tamsulosin
c) Tolazoline
d) Prazosin

4. Indicate the irreversible alfa receptor antagonist:
a) Tolazoline
b) Labetalol
c) Prazosin
d) Phenoxybenzamine

5. Which of the following drugs is an nonselective beta receptor antagonist?
a) Metoprolol
b) Atenolol
c) Propranolol
d) Acebutolol

6. Indicate the beta$_1$-selective antagonist:
a) Propranolol
b) Metoprolol
c) Carvedilol
d) Sotalol

7. Which of the following agents is a beta$_2$-selective antagonist?
a) Tolazolin
b) Pindolol
c) Ergotamin
d) Butoxamine

8. Indicate the beta adrenoreceptor antagonist, which has partial beta-agonist activity:
a) Propranolol
b) Metoprolol
c) Pindolol
d) Betaxolol

9. Which of the following drugs is a reversible nonselective alfa, beta antagonist?
a) Labetalol
b) Phentolamine
c) Metoprolol
d) Propranolol

10. Indicate the indirect-acting adrenoreceptor blocking drug:
a) Tolazoline
b) Reserpine
c) Carvedilol
d) Prazosin

11. The principal mechanism of action of adrenoreceptor antagonists is:
a) Reversible or irreversible interaction with adrenoreceptors
b) Depletion of the storage of catecholamines
c) Blockade of the amine reuptake pumps
d) Nonselective MAO inhibition

12. Characteristics of alfa-receptor antagonists include all of the following EXCEPT:
a) They cause a fall in peripheral resistance and blood pressure
b) They cause epinephrine reversal (convert a pressor response to a depressor response)
c) Bronchospasm
d) They may cause postural hypotension and reflex tachycardia

13. Which of the following drugs is an imidazoline derivative and a potent competitive antagonist at both alfa $_1$and alfa$_2$ receptors?

a) Prazosin
b) Labetalol
c) Phenoxybenzamine
d) Phentolamine

14. Characteristics of phentolamine include all of the following EXCEPT:
a) Reduction in peripheral resistance
b) Stimulation of responses to serotonin
c) Tachycardia
d) Stimulation of muscarinic, H_1 and H_2 histamine receptors

15. The principal mechanism of phentolamine-induced tachycardia is:
a) Antagonism of presynaptic alfa$_2$ receptors enhances norepinephrine release, which causes cardiac stimulation via unblocked beta receptors
b) Baroreflex mechanism
c) Direct effect on the heart by stimulation of beta$_1$ receptors
d) Inhibition of transmitter reuptake at noradrenergic synapses

16. Nonselective alfa-receptor antagonists are most useful in the treatment of:
a) Asthma
b) Cardiac arrhythmias
c) Pheochromocytoma
d) Chronic hypertension

17. The main reason for using alfa-receptor antagonists in the management of pheochromocytoma is:
a) Inhibition of the release of epinephrine from the adrenal medulla
b) Blockade of alfa $_2$ receptors on vascular smooth muscle results in epinephrine stimulation of unblocked alfa receptors
c) Direct interaction with and inhibition of beta$_2$ adrenoreceptors
d) Antagonism to the release of renin

18. Which of the following drugs is useful in the treatment of pheochromocytoma?
a) Phenylephrine
b) Propranolol
c) Phentolamine
d) Epinephrine

19. Indicate adrenoreceptor antagonist agents, which are used for the management of pheochromocytoma:
a) Selective beta$_2$-receptor antagonists

b) Nonselective beta-receptor antagonists
c) Indirect-acting adrenoreceptor antagonist drugs
d) Alfa-receptor antagonists

20. The principal adverse effects of phentolamine include all of the following EXCEPT:
a) Diarrhea
b) Bradycardia
c) Arrhythmias
d) Myocardial ischemia

21. Indicate the reversible nonselective alfa-receptor antagonist, which is an ergot derivative:
a) Ergotamine
b) Prazosin
c) Phenoxybenzamine
d) Carvedilol

22. Indicate an alfa-receptor antagonist, which binds covalently to alfa receptors, causing irreversible blockade of long duration (14-48 hours or longer):
a) Phentolamine
b) Phenoxybenzamine
c) Ergotamine
d) Prazosin

23. Compared with phentolamine, prazosin has all of the following features EXCEPT:
a) Irreversible blockade of alfa receptors
b) Highly selective for alfa$_1$ receptors
c) The relative absence of tachycardia
d) Persistent block of alfa$_1$ receptors

24. Which of the following statements is not correct?
a) There are at least three subtypes of alfa$_1$ receptors, designated alfa$_{1a}$, alfa$_{1b}$ and alfa$_{1d}$
b) ALFA$_{1a}$ subtype mediates prostate smooth muscle contraction
c) ALFA$_{1b}$ subtype mediates vascular smooth muscle contraction
d) ALFA$_{1a}$ subtype mediates both vascular and prostate smooth muscle contraction

25. Indicate an alfa $_1$ adrenoreceptor antagonist, which has great selectivity for alfa$_{1a}$ subtype:

a) Prazosin
b) Tamsulosin
c) Phenoxybenzamine
d) Phentolamine

26. Subtype-selective alfa₁receptor antagonists such as tamsulosin, terazosin, alfusosin are efficacious in:

a) Hyperthyroidism
b) Cardiac arrhythmias
c) Benign prostatic hyperplasia (BPH)
d) Asthma

27. Indicate an alfa receptor antagonist, which is an efficacious drug in the treatment of mild to moderate systemic hypertension:

a) Phentolamine
b) Tolazoline
c) Ergotamine
d) Prazosin

28. Which of the following alfa receptor antagonists is useful in reversing the intense local vasoconstriction caused by inadvertent infiltration of nor-epinephrine into subcutaneous tissue during intravenous administration?

a) Propranolol
b) Phentolamine
c) Tamsulosin
d) Ergotamine

29. Beta-blocking drugs-induced chronically lower blood pressure may be associated with theirs effects on:

a) The heart
b) The blood vessels
c) The renin-angiotensin system
d) All of the above

30. Characteristics of beta-blocking agents include all of the following EXCEPT:

a) They occupy beta receptors and competitively reduce receptor occupancy by catecholamines or other beta agonists
b) They do not cause hypotension in individuals with normal blood pressure
c) They induce depression and depleted stores of catecholamines
d) They can cause blockade in the atrioventricular node

31. Beta-receptor antagonists have all of the following cardiovascular effects EXCEPT:
a) The negative inotropic and chronotropic effects
b) Acute effects of these drugs include a fall in peripheral resistance
c) Vasoconstriction
d) Reduction of the release of renin

32. Beta-blocking agents have all of the following effects except:
a) Increase plasma concentrations of HDL and decrease of VLDL
b) Bronchoconstriction
c) Decrease of aqueous humor prodaction
d) "membrane-stabilizing" action

33. Beta-receptor antagonists cause:
a) Stimulation of lipolysis
b) Stimulation of gluconeogenesis
c) Inhibition of glycogenolysis
d) Stimulation of insulin secretion

34. Propranolol has all of the following cardiovascular effects EXCEPT:
a) It decreases cardiac work and oxygen demand
b) It reduces blood flow to the brain
c) It inhibits the renin secretion
d) It increases the atrioventricular nodal refractory period

35. Propranolol-induced adverse effects include all of the following EXCEPT:
a) Bronchoconstriction
b) "supersensitivity" of beta-adrenergic receptors (rapid withdrawal)
c) Hyperglycemia
d) Sedation, sleep disturbances, depression and sexual dysfunction

36. Propranolol is used in the treatment all of the following diseases EXCEPT:
a) Cardiovascular diseases
b) Hyperthyroidism
c) Migraine headache
d) Bronchial asthma

37. Metoprolol and atenolol:
a) Are members of the beta $_1$ -selective group
b) Are nonselective beta antagonists
c) Have intrinsic sympathomimetic activity
d) Have an anesthetic action

38. Which of the following beta receptor antagonists is preferable in patients with asthma, diabetes or peripheral vascular diseases?
a) Propranolol
b) Metoprolol
c) Nadolol
d) Timolol

39. Indicate a beta receptor antagonist, which has very long duration of action:
a) Metoprolol
b) Propranolol
c) Nadolol
d) Pindolol

40. Indicate a beta$_1$-selective receptor antagonist, which has very long duration of action:
a) Betaxolol
b) Sotalol
c) Nadolol
d) Metoprolol

41. Which of the following drugs is a nonselective beta-blocker without intrinsic sympathomimetic or local anesthetic activity and used for the treatment of life-threatening ventricular arrhythmias?
a) Propranolol
b) Oxprenolol
c) Sotalol
d) Atenolol

42. Indicate a beta receptor antagonist with intrinsic sympathomimetic activity:
a) Propranolol
b) Oxprenolol
c) Metoprolol
d) Carvedilol

43. Pindolol, oxprenolol have all of the following properties EXCEPT:
a) They are nonselective beta antagonists
b) They have no partial agonist activity
c) They are less likely to cause bradycardia and abnormalities in plasma lipids
d) They are effective in hypertension and angina

44. Which of the following drugs has both alfa$_1$-selective and beta-blocking effects?
a) Labetalol
b) Betaxolol
c) Propranolol
d) Timolol

45. Characteristics of carvedilol include all of the following EXCEPT:
a) It is a beta $_1$ -selective antagonist
b) It has both alfa$_1$-selective and beta-blocking effects
c) It attenuates oxygen free radical-initiated lipid peroxidation
d) It inhibits vascular smooth muscle mitogenesis

46. Indicate the adrenoreceptor antagonist drug, which is a rauwolfia alkaloid:
a) Prazosin
b) Propranolol
c) Reserpine
d) Phentolamine

47. Characteristics of reserpine include all of the following EXCEPT:
a) It inhibits the uptake of norepinephrine into vesicles and MAO
b) It decreases cardiac output, peripheral resistance and inhibits pressor reflexes
c) It may cause a transient sympathomimetic effect
d) It depletes stores of catecholamines and serotonin in the brain

48. Indicate a beta-blocker, which is particularly efficacious in thyroid storm:
a) Pindolol
b) Sotalol
c) Phentolamine
d) Propranolol

49. Beta-receptor blocking drugs are used in the treatment all of the following diseases EXCEPT:
a) Hypertension, ischemic heart disease, cardiac arrhythmias
b) Glaucoma
c) Pheochromocytoma
d) Hyperthyroidism

50. Beta-blocker-induced adverse effects include all of the following EXCEPT:

a) Bronchoconstriction

b) Depression of myocardial contractility and excitability

c) "supersensitivity" of beta-receptors associated with rapid withdrawal of drugs

d) Hyperglycemia

Answer Key

01-B 02-C 03-A 04-D 05-C 06-B 07-D 08-C 09-A 10-B 11-A 12-C 13-D 14-B 15-A 16-C 17-B 18-C 19-D 20-B 21-A 22-B 23-A 24-D 25-B 26-C 27-D 28-B 29-D 30-C 31-B 32-A 33-C 34-B 35-C 36-D 37-A 38-B 39-C 40-A 41-C 42-B 43-B 44-A 45-A 46-C 47-A 48-D 49-C 50-D

7. Hypnotic drugs

1. Hypnotic drugs are used to treat:
a) Psychosis
b) Sleep disorders
c) Narcolepsy
d) Parkinsonian disorders

2. Hypnotic drugs should:
a) Reduce anxiety and exert a calming effect
b) Induce absence of sensation
c) Produce drowsiness, encourage the onset and maintenance of sleep
d) Prevent mood swings in patients with bipolar affective disorders

3. Which of the following chemical agents are used in the treatment of insomnia?
a) Benzodiazepines
b) Imidazopyridines
c) Barbiturates
d) All of the above

4. Select a hypnotic drug, which is a benzodiazepine derivative:
a) Zolpidem
b) Flurazepam
c) Secobarbital
d) Phenobarbitone

5. Tick a hypnotic agent – a barbituric acid derivative:
a) Flurazepam
b) Zaleplon
c) Thyopental
d) Triazolam

6. Select a hypnotic drug, which is an imidazopyridine derivative:
a) Pentobarbital
b) Temazepam
c) Zolpidem
d) Chloral hydrate

7. Which of the following hypnotic agents is absorbed slowly?
a) Phenobarbital
b) Flurazepam
c) Triazolam
d) Temazepam

8. Which of the following barbiturates is an ultra-short-acting drug?
a) Secobarbital
b) Amobarbital
c) Thiopental
d) Phenobarbital

9. Indicate the barbituric acid derivative, which has 4-5 days elimination half-life:
a) Secobarbital
b) Thiopental
c) Phenobarbital
d) Amobarbital

10. Indicate the hypnotic benzodiazepine, which has the shortest elimination half-life:
a) Temazepam
b) Triazolam
c) Flurazepam
d) Diazepam

11. Which of the following hypnotic drugs is more likely to cause cumulative and residual effects?
a) Zolpidem
b) Temazepam
c) Phenobarbital
d) Triazolam

12. Which of the following hypnotic drugs increases the activity of hepatic drug-metabolizing enzyme systems?
a) Phenobarbital
b) Zolpidem
c) Flurazepam
d) Zaleplon

13. Hepatic microsomal drug-metabolizing enzyme induction leads to:
a) Barbiturate tolerance
b) Cumulative effects
c) Development of physical dependence
d) "hangover" effects

14. Indicate the hypnotic drug, which does not change hepatic drug-metabolizing enzyme activity?
a) Flurazepam
b) Zaleplon
c) Triazolam
d) All of the above

15. Barbiturates increase the rate of metabolism of:
a) Anticoagulants
b) Digitalis compounds
c) Glucocorticoids
d) All of the above

16. Which of the following agents inhibits hepatic metabolism of hypnotics?
a) Flumasenil
b) Cimetidin
c) Phenytoin
d) Theophylline

17. Which of the following factors can influence the biodisposition of hypnotic agents?
a) Alterations in the hepatic function resulting from a disease
b) Old age
c) Drug-induced increases or decreases in microsomal enzyme activities
d) All of the above

18. Which of the following hypnotics is preferred for elderly patients?
a) Phenobarbital
b) Flurozepam
c) Temazepam
d) Secobarbital

19. Which of the following hypnotics is preferred in patients with limited hepatic function?
a) Zolpidem
b) Amobarbital
c) Flurozepam
d) Pentobarbital

20. Indicate the mechanism of barbiturate action (at hypnotic doses):
a) Increasing the duration of the GABA-gated Cl^- channel openings
b) Directly activating the chloride channels
c) Increasing the frequency of Cl^- channel opening events
d) All of the above

21. Imidazopyridines are:
a) Partial agonists at brain $5\text{-}TH_{1A}$ receptors
b) Selective agonists of the BZ_1 (omega$_1$) subtype of BZ receptors
c) Competitive antagonists of BZ receptors
d) Nonselective agonists of both BZ_1 and BZ_2 receptor subtypes

22. Which of the following hypnotic agents is a positive allosteric modulator of $GABA_A$ receptor function?
a) Zaleplon
b) Flurazepam
c) Zolpidem
d) All of the above

23. Indicate a hypnotic drug - a selective agonist at the BZ_1 receptor subtype:
a) Flurazepam
b) Zolpidem
c) Triazolam
d) Flumazenil

24. Which of the following hypnotic agents is able to interact with both BZ_1 and BZ_2 receptor subtypes?
a) Zaleplon
b) Phenobarbital
c) Flurazepam
d) Zolpidem

25. Indicate the competitive antagonist of BZ receptors:
a) Flumazenil
b) Picrotoxin
c) Zolpidem
d) Temazepam

26. Flumazenil blocks the actions of:
a) Phenobarbital
b) Morphine
c) Zolpidem
d) Ethanol

27. Indicate the agent, which interferes with GABA binding:
a) Flurazepam
b) Bicuculline
c) Thiopental
d) Zolpidem

28. Which of the following agents blocks the chloride channel directly?
a) Secobarbital
b) Flumazenil
c) Zaleplon
d) Picrotoxin

29.Which of the following agents is preferred in the treatment of insomnia?
a) Barbiturates
b) Hypnotic benzodiazepines
c) Ethanol
d) Phenothiazide

30. Barbiturates are being replaced by hypnotic benzodiazepines because of:
a) Low therapeutic index
b) Suppression in REM sleep
c) High potential of physical dependence and abuse
d) All of the above

31. Which of the following benzodiazepines is used mainly for hypnosis?
a) Clonozepam
b) Lorazepam
c) Flurazepam
d) Midazolam

32. Indicate the main claim for an ideal hypnotic agent:
a) Rapid onset and sufficient duration of action
b) Minor effects on sleep patterns
c) Minimal "hangover" effects
d) All of the above

33.Which stage of sleep is responsible for the incidence of dreams?
a) REM sleep
b) Slow wave sleep
c) Stage 2NREM sleep
d) All of the above

34.During slow wave sleep (stage 3 and 4 NREM sleep):
a) Dreams occur
b) The secretion of adrenal steroids is at its highest
c) Somnambulism and nightmares occur
d) The secretion of somatotropin is at its lowest

35. All of the hypnotic drugs induce:
a) Increase the duration of REM sleep
b) Decrease the duration of REM sleep
c) Do not alter the duration of REM sleep
d) Increase the duration of slow wave sleep

36. Which of the following hypnotic drugs causes least suppression of REM sleep?
a) Flumazenil
b) Phenobarbital
c) Flurazepam
d) Secobarbital

37. Although the benzodiazepines continue to be the agents of choice for insomnia, they have:
a) The possibility of psychological and physiological dependence
b) Synergistic depression of CNS with other drugs (especially alcohol)
c) Residual drowsiness and daytime sedation
d) All of the above

38.Hypnotic benzodiazepines can cause:
a) A dose-dependent increase in both REM and slow wave sleep
b) Do not change sleep patterns
c) A dose-dependent decrease in both REM and slow wave sleep
d) A dose-dependent increase in REM sleep and decrease in slow wave sleep

39. Which one of the following hypnotic benzodiazepines is more likely to cause rebound insomnia?
a) Triazolam
b) Flurazepam
c) Temazepam
d) All of the above

40. Which of the following hypnotic benzodiazepines is more likely to cause "hangover" effects such as drowsiness, dysphoria, and mental or motor depression the following day?
a) Temazepam
b) Triazolam
c) Flurazepam
d) None of the above

41. Indicate the hypnotic drug, which binds selectively to the BZ $_1$ receptor subtype, facilitating GABAergic inhibition:
a) Thiopental
b) Zolpidem
c) Flurazepam
d) Phenobarbital

42. Which of the following statements is correct for zolpidem?
a) Causes minor effects on sleep patterns
b) The risk of development of tolerance and dependence is less than with the use of hypnotic benzodiazepines
c) Has minimal muscle relaxing and anticonvulsant effects
d) All of the above

43. Which agent exerts hypnotic activity with minimal muscle relaxing and anticonvulsant effects?
a) Flurazepam
b) Triazolam
c) Zaleplon
d) None of the above

44. Which of the following hypnotic drugs is used intravenously as anesthesia?
a) Thiopental
b) Phenobarbital
c) Flurazepam
d) Zolpidem

45. Indicate the usual cause of death due to overdose of hypnotics:
a) Depression of the medullar respiratory center
b) Hypothermia
c) Cerebral edema
d) Status epilepticus

46.Toxic doses of hypnotics may cause a circulatory collapse as a result of:
a) Blocking alfa adrenergic receptors
b) Increasing vagal tone
c) Action on the medullar vasomotor center
d) All of the above

Answer Key

01-B 02-C 03-D 04-B 05-C 06-C 07-D 08-C 09-C 10-B 11-C 12-A 13-A 14-D 15-D 16-B 17-D 18-C 19-A 20-A 21-B 22-D 23-B 24-C 25-A 26-C 27-B 28-D 29-B 30-D 31-C 32-D 33-A 34-C 35-B 36-C 37-D 38-C 39-A 40-C 41-B 42-D 43-C 44-A 45-A 46-C

8. Antiseizure drugs

1. The mechanism of action of antiseizure drugs is:
a) Enhancement of GABAergic (inhibitory) transmission
b) Diminution of excitatory (usually glutamatergic) transmission
c) Modification of ionic conductance
d) All of the above mechanisms

2. Which of the following antiseizure drugs produces enhancement of GABA-mediated inhibition?
a) Ethosuximide
b) Carbamazepine
c) Phenobarbital
d) Lamotrigine

3. Indicate an antiseizure drug, which has an impotent effect on the T-type calcium channels in thalamic neurons?
a) Carbamazepin
b) Lamotrigine
c) Ethosuximide
d) Phenytoin

4. Which of the following antiseizure drugs produces a voltage-dependent inactivation of sodium channels?
a) Lamotrigine
b) Carbamazepin
c) Phenytoin
d) All of the above

5. Indicate an antiseizure drug, inhibiting central effects of excitatory amino acids:
a) Ethosuximide
b) Lamotrigine
c) Diazepam
d) Tiagabine

6. The drug for partial and generalized tonic-clonic seizures is:
a) Carbamazepine

b) Valproate
c) Phenytoin
d) All of the above

7. Indicate an anti-absence drug:
a) Valproate
b) Phenobarbital
c) Carbamazepin
d) Phenytoin

8. The drug against myoclonic seizures is:
a) Primidone
b) Carbamazepine
c) Clonazepam
d) Phenytoin

9. The most effective drug for stopping generalized tonic-clonic status epilepticus in adults is:
a) Lamotrigine
b) Ethosuximide
c) Diazepam
d) Zonisamide

10. Select the appropriate consideration for phenytoin:
a) It blocks sodium channels
b) It binds to an allosteric regulatory site on the GABA-BZ receptor and prolongs the openings of the Cl⁻ channels
c) It effects on Ca^{2+} currents, reducing the low-threshold (T-type) current
d) It inhibits GABA-transaminase, which catalyzes the breakdown of GABA

11. Phenytoin is used in the treatment of:
a) Petit mal epilepsy
b) Grand mal epilepsy
c) Myoclonic seizures
d) All of the above

12. Dose-related adverse effect caused by phenytoin is:
a) Physical and psychological dependence
b) Exacerbated grand mal epilepsy
c) Gingival hyperplasia
d) Extrapyramidal symptoms

13. Granulocytopenia, gastrointestinal irritation, gingival hyperplasia, and facial hirsutism are possible adverse effects of:
a) Phenobarbital
b) Carbamazepin
c) Valproate
d) Phenytoin

14. The antiseizure drug, which induces hepatic microsomal enzymes, is:
a) Lamotrigine
b) Phenytoin
c) Valproate
d) None of the above

15. The drug of choice for partial seizures is:
a) Carbamazepin
b) Ethosuximide
c) Diazepam
d) Lamotrigine

16. The mechanism of action of carbamazepine appears to be similar to that of:
a) Benzodiazepines
b) Valproate
c) Phenytoin
d) Ethosuximide

17. Which of the following antiseizure drugs is also effective in treating trigeminal neuralgia?
a) Primidone
b) Topiramat
c) Carbamazepine
d) Lamotrigine

18. The most common dose-related adverse effects of carbamazepine are:
a) Diplopia, ataxia, and nausea
b) Gingival hyperplasia, hirsutism
c) Sedation, physical and psychological dependence
d) Hemeralopia, myasthenic syndrome

19. Indicate the drug of choice for status epilepticus in infants and children:
a) Phenobarbital sodium
b) Clonazepam

c) Ethosuximide

d) Phenytoin

20. Barbiturates are used in the emergency treatment of status epilepticus in infants and children because of:

a) They significantly decrease of oxygen utilization by the brain, protecting cerebral edema and ischemia

b) Short onset and duration of action

c) They do not have effect on sleep architecture

d) All of the above

21. Which of the following antiseizure drugs binds to an allosteric regulatory site on the GABA-BZ receptor, increases the duration of the Cl⁻channels openings:

a) Diazepam

b) Valproate

c) Phenobarbital

d) Topiramate

22. Adverse effect caused by phenobarbital is:

a) Physical and phychological dependence

b) Exacerbated petit mal epilepsy

c) Sedation

d) All of the above

23. Which of the following antiseizure drugs is a prodrug, metabolized to phenobarbital?

a) Phenytoin

b) Primidone

c) Felbamate

d) Vigabatrin

24. Indicate the antiseizure drug, which is a phenyltriazine derivative:

a) Phenobarbital

b) Clonazepam

c) Lamotrigine

d) Carbamazepin

25. Lamotrigine can be used in the treatment of:

a) Partial seizures

b) Absence

c) Myoclonic seizures

d) All of the above

26. The mechanism of vigabatrin's action is:
a) Direct action on the GABA receptor-chloride channel complex
b) Inhibition of GABA aminotransferase
c) NMDA receptor blockade via the glycine binding site
d) Inhibition of GABA neuronal reuptake from synapses

27. Indicate an irreversible inhibitor of GABA aminotransferase (GABA-T):
a) Diazepam
b) Phenobarbital
c) Vigabatrin
d) Felbamate

28. Tiagabine:
a) Blocks neuronal and glial reuptake of GABA from synapses
b) Inhibits GABA-T, which catalyzed the breakdown of GABA
c) Blocks the T-type Ca^{2+} channels
d) Inhibits glutamate transmission at AMPA/kainate receptors

29. The mechanism of both topiramate and felbamate action is:
a) Reduction of excitatory glutamatergic neurotransmission
b) Inhibition of voltage sensitive Na^+ channels
c) Potentiation of GABAergic neuronal transmission
d) All of the above

30. The drug of choice in the treatment of petit mal (absence seizures) is:
a) Phenytoin
b) Ethosuximide
c) Phenobarbital
d) Carbamazepin

31. The dose-related adverse effect of ethosuximide is:
a) Gastrointestinal reactions, such as anorexia, pain, nausea and vomiting
b) Exacerbated grand mal epilepsy
c) Transient lethargy or fatigue
d) All of the above

32. Valproate is very effective against:
a) Absence seizures
b) Myoclonic seizures
c) Generalized tonic-clonic seizures
d) All of the above

33. The drug of choice in the treatment of myoclonic seizures is:
a) Valproate
b) Phenobarbital
c) Phenytoin
d) Felbamate

34. The reason for preferring ethosuximide to valproate for uncomplicated absence seizures is:
a) More effective
b) Valproate's idiosyncratic hepatotoxicity
c) Greater CNS depressant activity
d) All of the above

35. The mechanism of valproate action is:
a) Facilitation glutamic acid decarboxylase, the enzyme responsible for GABA synthesis and inhibition of GABA-aminotransferase, the enzyme responsible for the breakdown of GABA (enhance GABA accumulation)
b) Inhibition of voltage sensitive Na^+ channels
c) Inhibition of low threshold (T-type) Ca^{2+} channels
d) All of the above

36. Indicate the antiseizure drug, which is a sulfonamide derivative, blocking Na^+ channels and having additional ability to inhibit T-type Ca^{2+} channels:
a) Tiagabine
b) Zonisamide
c) Ethosuximide
d) Primidone

37. Indicate the antiseizure drug – a benzodiazepine receptor agonist:
a) Phenobarbital
b) Phenytoin
c) Carbamazepine
d) Lorazepam

38. Which of the following antiseizure drugs acts directly on the GABA receptor-chloride channel complex?
a) Vigabatrin
b) Diazepam
c) Gabapentin
d) Valproate

39. Benzodiazepine's uselfulness is limited by:
a) Tolerance
b) Atropine-like symptoms
c) Psychotic episodes
d) Myasthenic syndrome

40. A long-acting drug against both absence and myoclonic seizures is:
a) Primidone
b) Carbamazepine
c) Clonazepam
d) Phenytoin

41. Which of the following antiseizure drugs may produce teratogenicity?
a) Phenytoin
b) Valproate
c) Topiramate
d) All of the above

42. The most dangerous effect of antiseizure drugs after large overdoses is:
a) Respiratory depression
b) Gastrointestinal irritation
c) Alopecia
d) Sedation

Answer Key

01-D 02-C 03-C 04-D 05-B 06-D 07-A 08-C 09-C 10-A 11-B 12-C 13-D 14-A 15-A 16-C 17-C 18-A 19-A 20-A 21-C 22-D 23-B 24-C 25-D 26-B 27-C 28-A 29-D 30-B 31-D 32-D 33-A 34-B 35-D 36-B 37-D 38-B 39-A 40-C 41-D 42-A

9. Antiparkinsonian agents

1. Which neurons are involved in parkinsonism?
a) Cholinergic neurons
b) GABAergic neurons
c) Dopaminergic neurons
d) All of the above

2. The pathophysiologic basis for antiparkinsonism therapy is:
a) A selective loss of dopaminergic neurons
b) The loss of some cholinergic neurons
c) The loss of the GABAergic cells
d) The loss of glutamatergic neurons

3. Which of the following neurotransmitters is involved in Parkinson's disease?
a) Acetylcholine
b) Glutamate
c) Dopamine
d) All of the above

4. Principal aim for treatment of Parkinsonian disorders is:
a) To restore the normal balance of cholinergic and dopaminergic influences on the basal ganglia with antimuscarinic drugs
b) To restore dopaminergic activity with levodopa and dopamine agonists
c) To decrease glutamatergic activity with glutamate antagonists
d) All of the above

5. Indicate the drug that induces parkinsonian syndromes:
a) Chlorpromazine
b) Diazepam
c) Triazolam
d) Carbamazepine

6. Which of the following drugs is used in the treatment of Parkinsonian disorders?
a) Phenytoin
b) Selegiline

c) Haloperidol
d) Fluoxetine

7. Select the agent, which is preferred in the treatment of the drug-induced form of parkinsonism:
a) Levodopa
b) Bromocriptine
c) Benztropine
d) Dopamine

8. Which of the following agents is the precursor of dopamine?
a) Bromocriptine
b) Levodopa
c) Selegiline
d) Amantadine

9. The main reason for giving levodopa, the precursor of dopamine, instead of dopamine is:
a) Dopamine does not cross the blood-brain barrier
b) Dopamine may induce acute psychotic reactions
c) Dopamine is intensively metabolized in humans
d) All of the above

10. Indicate a peripheral dopa decarboxylase inhibitor:
a) Tolcapone
b) Clozapine
c) Carbidopa
d) Selegiline

11. The mechanism of carbidopa's action is:
a) Stimulating the synthesis, release, or reuptake of dopamine
b) Inhibition of dopa decarboxilase
c) Stimulating dopamine receptors
d) Selective inhibition of catecol-O-methyltransferase

12. When carbidopa and levodopa are given concomitantly:
a) Levodopa blood levels are increased, and drug half-life is lengthened
b) The dose of levodopa can be significantly reduced (by 75%), also reducing toxic side effects
c) A shorter latency period precedes the occurrence of beneficial effects
d) All of the above

13. Which of the following preparations combines carbidopa and levodopa in a fixed proportion?
a) Selegiline
b) Sinemet
c) Tolkapone
d) Biperiden

14. Which of the following statements is correct for levodopa?
a) Tolerance to both beneficial and adverse effects develops gradually
b) Levodopa is most effective in the first 2-5 years of treatment
c) After 5 years of therapy, patients have dose-related dyskinesias, inadequate response or toxicity
d) All of the above

15. Gastrointestinal irritation, cardiovascular effects, including tachycardia, arrhythmias, and orthostatic hypotension, mental disturbances, and withdrawal are possible adverse effects of:
a) Amantadine
b) Benztropine
c) Levodopa
d) Selegiline

16.Which of the following agents is the most helpful in counteracting the behavioral complications of levodopa?
a) Tolkapone
b) Clozapine
c) Carbidopa
d) Pergolide

17. Which of the following vitamins reduces the beneficial effects of levodopa by enhancing its extracerebral metabolism?
a) Pyridoxine
b) Thiamine
c) Tocopherol
d) Riboflavin

18. Which of the following drugs antagonizes the effects of levodopa because it leads to a junctional blockade of dopamine action?
a) Reserpine
b) Haloperidol
c) Chlorpromazine
d) All of the above

19. Levodopa should not be given to patients taking:
a) Bromocriptine
b) Monoamine oxydase A inhibitors
c) Carbidopa
d) Nonselective beta-adrenergic antagonists

20. Indicate D_2 receptor agonist with antiparkinsonian activity:
a) Sinemet
b) Levodopa
c) Bromocriptine
d) Selegiline

21. Which of the following antiparkinsonian drugs has also been used to treat hyperprolactinemia?
a) Benztropine
b) Bromocriptine
c) Amantadine
d) Levodopa

22. Indicate a selective inhibitor of monoamine oxidase B:
a) Levodopa
b) Amantadine
c) Tolcapone
d) Selegiline

23. Which of the following statements is correct?
a) MAO-A metabolizes dopamine; MAO-B metabolizes serotonin
b) MAO-A metabolizes norepinephrine and dopamine; MAO-B metabolizes serotonin
c) MAO-A metabolizes norepinephrine and serotonin; MAO-B metabolizes dopamine
d) MAO-A metabolizes dopamine; MAO-B metabolizes norepinephrine and serotonin

24. The main reason for avoiding the combined administration of levodopa and an inhibitor of both forms of monoamine oxidase is:
a) Respiratory depression
b) Hypertensive emergency
c) Acute psychotic reactions
d) Cardiovascular collapse and CNS depression

25. Indicate selective catechol-O-methyltransferase inhibitor, which prolongs the action of levodopa by diminishing its peripheral metabolism:
a) Carbidopa
b) Clozapine
c) Tolcapone
d) Rasagiline

26. Which of the following antiparkinsonian drugs is an antiviral agent used in the prophylaxis of influenza A $_2$?
a) Selegiline
b) Sinemet
c) Pergolide
d) Amantadine

27.The mechanism of amantadine action is :
a) Stimulating the glutamatergic neurotransmission
b) Blocking the excitatory cholinergic system
c) Inhibition of dopa decarboxilase
d) Selective inhibition of catechol-O-methyltransferase

28.Which of the following antiparkinsonis drugs anticholinergic agent?
a) Amantadine
b) Selegilin
c) Trihexyphenidyl
d) Bromocriptine

29. Mental confusion and hallucinations, peripheral atropine-like toxicity (e.g. Cycloplegia, tachycardia, urinary retention, and constipation) are possible adverse effects of:
a) Sinemet
b) Benztropine
c) Tolkapone
d) Bromocriptine

30. Indicate the antiparkinsonism drug which should be avoided in patients with glaucoma:
a) Selegilin
b) Levodopa
c) Bromocriptine
d) Trihexyphenidyl

Answer Key

01-D,02-A, 03-D, 04-D,05-A,06-B,07-C,08-B,09-A,10-C,11-B,12-D,13-B,14-D, 15-C,16-B,17-A,18-D,19-B,20-C,21-B,22-D,23-C,24-B,25-C,26-D,27-A,28-C,29-B, 30-D

10.Ethyl alcohol

1. Alcohol may cause:
a) CNS depression
b) Vasodilatation
c) Hypoglycemia
d) All of the above

2. Alcohol:
a) Increases body temperature
b) Decreases body heat loss
c) Increases body heat loss
d) Does not affect body temperature

3. The most common medical complication of alcohol abuse is:
a) Liver failure including liver cirrhosis
b) Tolerance and physical dependence
c) Generalized symmetric peripheral nerve injury, ataxia and dementia
d) All of the above

4. Effect of moderate consumption of alcohol on plasma lipoproteins is:
a) Raising serum levels of high-density lipoproteins
b) Increasing serum concentration of low-density lipoproteins
c) Decreasing the concentration of high-density lipoproteins
d) Raising serum levels of very low-density lipoproteins

5. Which of the following metabolic alterations may be associated with chronic alcohol abuse?
a) Hyperglycemia
b) Increased serum concentration of phosphate
c) Severe loss of potassium and magnesium
d) Decreased serum concentration of sodium

6. Alcohol potentiates:
a) SNS depressants
b) Vasodilatators
c) Hypoglycemic agents
d) All of the above

7. Which of the following drugs is most commonly used for causing a noxious reaction to alcohol by blocking its metabolism?
a) Naltrexone
b) Disulfiram
c) Diazepam
d) Morphine

8. Which of the following agents is an inhibitor of aldehyde dehydrogenase?
a) Fomepizole
b) Ethanol
c) Disulfiram
d) Naltrexone

9. Indicate the drug, which alters brain responses to alcohol:
a) Naltrexone
b) Disulfiram
c) Amphetamine
d) Chlorpromazine

10.Which of the following agents is an opioid antagonist?
a) Amphetamine
b) Naltrexone
c) Morphine
d) Disulfiram

11. Alcohol causes an acute increase in the local concentrations of:
a) Dopamine
b) Opioid
c) Serotonine
d) All of the above

12. Management of alcohol withdrawal syndrome contains:
a) Restoration of potassium, magnesium and phosphate balance
b) Thiamine therapy
c) Substituting a long-acting sedative-hypnotic drug for alcohol
d) All of the above

13. Indicate the drug, which decreases the craving for alcohol or blunts pleasurable "high" that comes with renewed drinking:
a) Disulfiram
b) Amphetamine

c) Naltrexone

d) Diazepam

14. The symptoms resulting from the combination of disulfiram and alcohol are:

a) Hypertensive crisis leading to cerebral ischemia and edema

b) Nausea, vomiting

c) Respiratory depression and seizures

d) Acute psychotic reactions

15. The combination of disulfiram and ethanol leads to accumulation of:

a) Formaldehyde

b) Acetate

c) Formic acid

d) Acetaldehyde

16. Indicate the "specific" modality of treatment for severe methanol poisoning:

a) Dialysis to enhance removal of methanol

b) Alkalinization to counteract metabolic acidosis

c) Suppression of metabolism by alcohol dehydrogenase to toxic products

d) All of the above

17. Which of the following agents may be used as an antidote for ethylene glycol and methanol poisoning?

a) Disulfiram

b) Fomepizol

c) Naltrexone

d) Amphetamine

18. The principal mechanism of fomepizol action is associated with inhibition of:

a) Aldehyde dehydrogenase

b) Acethylholinesterase

c) Alcohol dehydrogenase

d) Monoamine oxidase

Answer Key

01-D,02-C,03-D,04-A,05-C,06-D,07-B,08-C,09-A,10-B,11-D,12-D,13-C,14-B,15-D,16-D,17-B,18-C

11.Narcotic analgesics

1. Narcotics analgesics should:
a) Relieve severe pain
b) Induce loss of sensation
c) Reduce anxiety and exert a calming effect
d) Induce a stupor or somnolent state

2. Second-order pain is:
a) Sharp, well-localized pain
b) Dull, burning pain
c) Associated with fine myelinated A-delta fibers
d) Effectively reduced by non-narcotic analgesics

3. Chemical mediators in the nociceptive pathway are all of the following EXCEPT:
a) Enkephalins
b) Kinins
c) Prostaglandins
d) Substance P

4. Indicate the chemical mediator in the antinociceptive descending pathways:
a) BETA-endorphin
b) Met- and leu-enkephalin
c) Dynorphin
d) All of the above

5. Which of the following mediators is found mainly in long descending pathways from the midbrain to the dorsal horn?
a) Prostaglandin E
b) Dynorphin
c) Enkephalin
d) Glutamate

6. Select the brain and spinal cord regions, which are involved in the transmission of pain?
a) The limbic system, including the amygdaloidal nucleus and the hypothalamus
b) The ventral and medial parts of the thalamus

c) The substantia gelatinosa
d) All of the above

7. Mu (μ) receptors are associated with:
a) Analgesia, euphoria, respiratory depression, physical dependence
b) Spinal analgesia, mydriasis, sedation, physical dependence
c) Dysphoria, hallucinations, respiratory and vasomotor stimulation
d) Analgesia, euphoria, respiratory stimulation, physical dependence

8. Which of the following opioid receptor types is responsible for euphoria and respiratory depression?
a) Kappa-receptors
b) Delta-receptors
c) Mu-receptors
d) All of the above

9. Indicate the opioid receptor type, which is responsible for dysphoria and vasomotor stimulation:
a) Kappa-receptors
b) Delta-receptors
c) Mu-receptors
d) All of the above

10. Kappa and delta agonists:
a) Inhibit postsynaptic neurons by opening K^+ channels
b) Close a voltage-gated Ca^{2+} channels on presynaptic nerve terminals
c) Both a and b
d) Inhibit of arachidonate cyclooxygenase in CNS

11. Which of the following supraspinal structures is implicated in pain-modulating descending pathways?
a) The midbrain periaqueductal gray
b) The hypothalamus
c) The aria postrema
d) The limbic cortex

12. Indicate the neurons, which are located in the locus ceruleus or the lateral tegmental area of the reticular formation:
a) Dopaminergic
b) Serotoninergic
c) Nonadrenergic
d) Gabaergic

13. Which of the following analgesics is a phenanthrene derivative?
a) Fentanyl
b) Morphine
c) Methadone
d) Pentazocine

14. Tick narcotic analgesic, which is a phenylpiperidine derivative:
a) Codeine
b) Dezocine
c) Fentanyl
d) Buprenorphine

15. Which of the following opioid analgesics is a strong mu receptor agonist?
a) Naloxone
b) Morphine
c) Pentazocine
d) Buprenorphine

16. Indicate the narcotic analgesic, which is a natural agonist:
a) Meperidine
b) Fentanyl
c) Morphine
d) Naloxone

17. Select the narcotic analgesic, which is an antagonist or partial mu receptor agonist:
a) Fentanyl
b) Pentazocine
c) Codeine
d) Methadone

18. Which of the following agents is a full antagonist of opioid receptors?
a) Meperidine
b) Buprenorphine
c) Naloxone
d) Butorphanol

19. The principal central nervous system effect of the opioid analgesics with affinity for a mu receptor is:
a) Analgesia
b) Respiratory depression

c) Euphoria

d) All of the above

20. Which of the following opioid analgesics can produce dysphoria, anxiety and hallucinations?

a) Morphine

b) Fentanyl

c) Pentazocine

d) Methadone

21. Indicate the opioid analgesic, which has 80 times analgesic potency and respiratory depressant properties of morphine, and is more effective than morphine in maintaining hemodynamic stability?

a) Fentanyl

b) Pentazocine

c) Meperidine

d) Nalmefene

22. Which of the following opioid analgesics is used in combination with droperidol in neuroleptanalgesia?

a) Morphine

b) Buprenorphine

c) Fentanyl

d) Morphine

23. Fentanyl can produce significant respiratory depression by:

a) Inhibiting brain stem respiratory mechanisms

b) Suppression of the cough reflex leading to airway obstruction

c) Development of truncal rigidity

d) Both a and c

24. Most strong mu receptor agonists cause:

a) Hypertension

b) Increasing the pulmonary arterial pressure and myocardial work

c) Cerebral vasodilatation, causing an increase in intracranial pressure

d) All of the above

25. Which of the following opioid analgesics can produce an increase in the pulmonary arterial pressure and myocardial work?

a) Morphine

b) Pentazocine

c) Meperidine

d) Methadone

26. Morphine causes the following effects EXCEPT:
a) Constipation
b) Dilatation of the biliary duct
c) Urinary retention
d) Bronchiolar constriction

27. Therapeutic doses of the opioid analgesics:
a) Decrease body temperature
b) Increase body temperature
c) Decrease body heat loss
d) Do not affect body temperature

28. Which of the following opioid analgesics is used in obstetric labor?
a) Fentanyl
b) Pentazocine
c) Meperidine
d) Buprenorphine

29. Indicate the opioid analgesic, which is used for relieving the acute, severe pain of renal colic:
a) Morphine
b) Naloxone
c) Methadone
d) Meperidine

30. Which of the following opioid analgesics is used in the treatment of acute pulmonary edema?
a) Morphine
b) Codeine
c) Fentanyl
d) Loperamide

31. The relief produced by intravenous morphine in dyspnea from pulmonary edema is associated with reduced:
a) Perception of shortness of breath
b) Patient anxiety
c) Cardiac preload (reduced venous tone) and afterload (decreased peripheral resistance)
d) All of the above

32. Rhinorrhea, lacrimation, chills, gooseflesh, hyperventilation, hyperthermia, mydriasis, muscular aches, vomiting, diarrhea, anxiety, and hostility are effects of:
a) Tolerance
b) Opioid overdosage
c) Drug interactions between opioid analgesics and sedative-hypnotics
d) Abstinence syndrome

33. The diagnostic triad of opioid overdosage is:
a) Mydriasis, coma and hyperventilation
b) Coma, depressed respiration and miosis
c) Mydriasis, chills and abdominal cramps
d) Miosis, tremor and vomiting

33. Which of the following opioid agents is used in the treatment of acute opioid overdose?
a) Pentazocine
b) Methadone
c) Naloxone
d) Remifentanyl

34. Indicate the pure opioid antagonist, which has a half-life of 10 hours:
a) Naloxone
b) Naltrexone
c) Tramadol
d) Pentazocine

36. In contrast to morphine, methadone:
a) Causes tolerance and physical dependence more slowly
b) Is more effective orally
c) Withdrawal is less severe, although more prolonged
d) All of the above

37. Which of the following opioid analgesics is a partial mu receptor agonist?
a) Morphine
b) Methadone
c) Buprenorphine
d) Sufentanyl

38. Indicate a partial mu receptor agonist, which has 20-60 times analgesic potency of morphine, and a longer duration of action:

a) Pentazocine

b) Buprenorphine
c) Nalbuphine
d) Naltrexone

39. Which of the following opioid analgesics is a strong kappa receptor agonist and a mu receptor antagonist?

a) Naltrexone
b) Methadone
c) Nalbuphine
d) Buprenorphine

40. Which of the following drugs has weak mu agonist effects and inhibitory action on norepinephrine and serotonin reuptake in the CNS?

a) Loperamide
b) Tramadol
c) Fluoxetine
d) Butorphanol

Answer Key

01-A,02-B,03-A 04-D 05-C,06-D,07-A,08-C,09-A,10-B,11-A,12-C,13-B,14-C,15-B,16-C,17-B,18-C,19-D,20-C,21-A,22-C,23-D,24-C,25-B,26-B,27-A,28-C,29-D,30-A,31-D,32-D,33-D,33-B,34-C,35-B,36-D,37-C,38-B,39-C,40-B

12. Non-narcotic analgesics

1. Non-narcotic analgesics are mainly effective against pain associated with:
a) Inflammation or tissue damage
b) Trauma
c) Myocardial infarction
d) Surgery

2. Non-narcotic agents cause:
a) Respiratory depression
b) Antipyretic effect
c) Euphoria
d) Physical dependence

3. Non-narcotic analgesics are all of the following drugs EXCEPT:
a) Paracetamol
b) Acetylsalicylic acid
c) Butorphanol
d) Ketorolac

4. Select the non-narcotic drug, which is a paraaminophenol derivative:
a) Analgin
b) Aspirin
c) Baclophen
d) Paracetamol

5. Which of the following non-narcotic agents is salicylic acid derivative?
a) Phenylbutazone
b) Ketamine
c) Aspirin
d) Tramadol

6. Tick pirazolone derivative:
a) Methylsalicylate
b) Analgin
c) Paracetamol
d) Ketoralac

7. Which one of the following non-narcotic agents inhibits mainly cyclooxygenase (COX) in CNS?
a) Paracetamol
b) Ketorolac
c) Acetylsalicylic acid
d) Ibuprofen

8. Most of non-narcotic analgetics have:
a) Anti-inflammatory effect
b) Analgesic effect
c) Antipyretic effect
d) All of the above

9. Indicate the non-narcotic analgesic, which lacks an anti-inflammatory effect:
a) Naloxone
b) Paracetamol
c) Metamizole
d) Aspirin

10. Correct statements concerning aspirin include all of the following EXCEPT:
a) It inhibits mainly peripheral COX
b) It does not have an anti-inflammatory effect
c) It inhibits platelet aggregation
d) It stimulates respiration by a direct action on the respiratory center

11. For which of the following conditions could aspirin be used prophylactically?
a) Noncardiogenic pulmonary edema
b) Peptic ulcers
c) Thromboembolism
d) Metabolic acidosis

12. All of the following are undesirable effects of aspirin EXCEPT:
a) Gastritis with focal erosions
b) Tolerance and physical addiction
c) Bleeding due to a decrease of platelet aggregation
d) Reversible renal insufficiency

13. Characteristic findinds of salicylism include:

a) Headache, mental confusion and drowsiness

b) Tinnitus and difficulty in hearing

c) Hyperthermia, sweating, thirst, hyperventilation, vomiting and diarrhea

d) All of the above

14. Analgin usefulness is limited by:

a) Agranulocytosis

b) Erosions and gastric bleeding

c) Methemoglobinemia

d) Hearing impairment

15. Methemoglobinemia is possible adverse effect of:

a) Aspirin

b) Paracetamol

c) Analgin

d) Ketorolac

16. Correct the statements concerning ketorolac include all of the following EXCEPT:

a) It inhibits COX

b) It is as effective as morphine for a short-term relief from moderate to severe pain

c) It has a high potential for physical dependence and abuse

d) It does not produce respiratory depression

17. Indicate the nonopioid agent of central effect with analgesic activity:

a) Reserpine

b) Propranolol

c) Clopheline

d) Prazosin

18. Select the antiseizure drug with an analgesic component of effect:

a) Carbamazepine

b) Ethosuximide

c) Phenytoin

d) Clonazepam

19. Which of the following nonopioid agents is an antidepressant with analgesic activity?
a) Fluoxetine
b) Moclobemide
c) Tranylcypramine
d) Amitriptyline

20. Tick mixed (opioid/non-opioid) agent:
 a) Paracetamol
b) Tramadol
c) Sodium valproate
d) Butorphanol

Answer Key

01-A,02-B,03-C,04-D,05-C,06-B,07-A,08-D,09-B,10-B,11-C12-B,13-D,14-A,15-B,16-C,17-C,18-A,19-D,20-B

13. Antipsychotic agents

1. Neuroleptics are used to treat:
a) Neurosis
b) Psychosis
c) Narcolepsy
d) Parkinsonian disorders

2. Most antipsychotic drugs:
a) Strongly block postsynaptic d $_2$ receptor
b) Stimulate postsynaptic D_2receptor
c) Block NMDA receptor
d) Stimulate 5-HT$_2$receptor

3. Which of the following dopaminergic systems is most closely related to behavior?
a) The hypothalamic-pituitary system
b) The extrapyramidal system
c) The mesolimbic and mesofrontal systems
d) The chemoreceptor trigger zone of the medulla

4. Hyperprolactinemia is caused by blockade of dopamine in:
a) The chemoreceptor trigger zone of the medulla
b) The pituitary
c) The extrapiramidal system
d) The mesolimbic and mesofrontal systems

5. Parkinsonian symptoms and tarditive dyskinesia are caused by blockade dopamine in:
a) The nigrostriatal system
b) The mesolimbic and mesofrontal systems
c) The chemoreceptor trigger zone of the medulla
d) The tuberoinfundibular system

6. Extrapyramidal reactions can be treated by:
a) Levodopa
b) Benztropine mesylate
c) Bromocriptine
d) Dopamine

7. Which of the following statements is true?
a) D_1 postsynaptic receptors are located in striatum
b) D_2 pre- and postsynaptic receptors are located in striatum and limbic areas
c) D_4 postsynaptic receptors are located in frontal cortex, mesolimbic system
d) All of the above

8. Which of the following antipsychotic drugs is typical?
a) Clozapine
b) Quetiapine
c) Haloperidol
d) Olanzapine

9. Indicate the atypical antipsychotic drug:
a) Haloperidol
b) Clozapine
c) Thioridazine
d) Thiothixene

10. Atypical antipsychotic agents (such as clozapine) differ from typical ones:
a) In reduced risks of extrapyramidal system dysfunction and tardive dyscinesia
b) In having low affinity for D_1 and D_2 dopamine receptors
c) In having high affinity for D_4 dopamine receptors
d) All of the above

11. Tardive dyskinesia is the result of:
a) Degeneration of dopaminergic and cholinergic fibers
b) Hyperactive dopaminergic state in the presence of dopamine blockers
c) Degeneration of histaminergic fibers
d) Supersensitivity of cholinergic receptors in the caudate-putamen

12. Which of the following antipsychotic drugs has high affinity for D_4 and 5-HT_2 receptors?
a) Clozapine
b) Fluphenazine
c) Thioridazine
d) Haloperidole

13. Indicate the antipsychotic drug, which is a phenothiazine aliphatic derivative:
a) Thiothixene
b) Risperidone
c) Chlorpromazine
d) Clozapine

13. Indicate the antipsychotic drug, which is a butyrophenone derivative :
a) Droperidol
b) Thioridazine
c) Sertindole
d) Fluphenazine

15. Indicate the antipsychotic drug, which is a thioxanthene derivative:
a) Haloperidol
b) Clozapine
c) Chlorpromazine
d) Thiothixene

16. Indicate the antipsychotic agent – a dibenzodiazepine derivative:
a) Fluphenazine
b) Clozapine
c) Risperidone
d) Droperidol

17. The strong antiemetic effect of the phenothiazine derivatives is due to dopamine receptor blockade:
a) In the chemoreceptor trigger zone of the medulla
b) Of the receptors in the stomach
c) The medullar vomiting centre
d) All of the above

18. Phenothiazine derivatives are able to:
a) Alter temperature-regulating mechanisms producing hypothermia
b) Decrease levels of prolactin
c) Increase corticotrophin release and secretion of pituitary growth hormone
d) Decrease appetite and weight

19. Most phenothiazine derivatives have:
a) Antihistaminic activity
b) Anticholinergic activity
c) Antidopaminergic activity
d) All of the above

20. Indicate the antipsychotic drug having significant peripheral alpha-adrenergic blocking activity:
a) Haloperidol
b) Chlorpromazine
c) Clozapine
d) Risperidone

21. Indicate the antipsychotic drug having a muscarinic-cholinergic blocking activity:
a) Chlorpromazine
b) Clorprothixene
c) Risperidone
d) Haloperidol

22. Indicate the antipsychotic drug having H_1-antihistaminic activity:
a) Clozapine
b) Chlorpromazine
c) Olanzapine
d) All of the above

23. Parkinson's syndrome, acute dystonic reactions, tardive dyskinesia, antimuscarinic actions, orthostatic hypotension, galactorrhea are possible adverse effects of:
a) Haloperidol
b) Clozapine
c) Chlorpromazine
d) Risperidone

24. Orthostatic hypotension can occur as a result of:
a) The central action of phenothiazines
b) Inhibition of norepinephrine uptake mechanisms
c) Alpha adrenoreceptor blockade
d) All of the above

25. Adverse peripheral effects, such as loss of accommodation, dry mouth, tachycardia, urinary retention, constipation are related to:
a) Alpha adrenoreceptor blockade
b) Muscarinic cholinoreceptor blockade
c) Supersesitivity of the dopamine receptor
d) Dopamine receptor blockade

26. Which of the following phenothiazine derivatives is a potent local anesthetic?
a) Fluphenazine
b) Thioridazine
c) Chlorpromazine
d) None of the above

27. Which of the following phenothiazine derivatives may produce cardiac toxicity, including ventricular arrhythmias, cardiac conduction block, and sudden death?
a) Thioridazine
b) Chlorpromazine
c) Perphenazine
d) Fluphenazine

28. Which of the following antipsychotic agents is preferable in patients with coronary and cerebrovascular disease?
a) Chlorpromazine
b) Fluphenazine
c) Haloperidol
d) Perphenazine

29. Which of the following antipsychotic agents is used in combination with an opioid drug fentanyl in neuroleptanalgesia?
a) Haloperidol
b) Droperidol
c) Chlorpromazine
d) Clozapine

30. The mechanism of haloperidol antipsychotic action is:
a) Blocking D_2receptors
b) Central alpha-adrenergic blocking
c) Inhibition of norepinephrine uptake mechanisms
d) All of the above

31. Which of the following statements is correct for clozapine?
a) Has potent anticholinergic activity
b) Has high affinity for $D_1$and D_2dopamine receptors
c) Produces significant extrapyramidal toxicity
d) Is related to typical antipsychotic agents

32. Which of the following antipsychotic drugs has the high risk of potentially fatal agranulocytosis and risk of seizures at high doses ?

a) Haloperidol
b) Risperidone
c) Clozapine
d) Chlorpromazine

33. Which of the following antipsychotic drugs has high affinity for D_2 and 5-HT_2 receptors?
a) Droperidol
b) Clozapine
c) Thiothixene
d) Risperidone

34. Lithium carbonate is useful in the treatment of:
a) Petit mal seizures
b) Bipolar disorder
c) Neurosis
d) Trigeminal neuralgia

35. The drug of choice for manic-depressive psychosis is:
a) Imipramine
b) Chlordiazepoxide
c) Isocarboxazid
d) Lithium carbonate

36. The lithium mode of action is:
a) Effect on electrolytes and ion transport
b) Effect on neurotransmitters
c) Effect on second messengers
d) All of the above

37. Which of the following statements is correct for lithium?
a) Stimulate dopamine and beta-adrenergic receptors
b) Decrease catecholamine-related activity
c) Stimulate the development of dopamine receptor supersensitivity
d) Decrease cholinergic activity

38. Which of the following adverse effects is associated with lithium treatment?

a) Cardiovascular anomalies in the newborn

b) Thyroid enlargement

c) Nephrogenic diabetes insipidus

d) All of the above

Answer Key

01-B,02-A,03-C,04-B,05-A,06-B,07-D,08-C,09-B,10-D,11-B,12-A,13-C,14-A,15-D,16-B,17-D,18-A,19-D,20-B,21-A,22-D,23-C,24-D,25-B,26-C,27-A,28-C,29-B,30-D,31-A,32-C,33-D,34-B,35-D,36-D,37-B,38-D

14. Antidepressant agents

1. The principal mechanism of action of antidepressant agents is:
a) Stabilization of dopamine and beta-adrenergic receptors
b) Inhibition of the storage of serotonin and epinephrine in the vesicles of presynaptic nerve endings
c) Blocking epinephrine or serotonin reuptake pumps
d) Stimulation of alfa$_2$-norepinephrine receptors

2. Which of the following agents is related to tricyclic antidepressants?
a) Nefazodon
b) Amitriptyline
c) Fluoxetine
d) Isocarboxazid

3. Indicate the second-generation heterocyclic drug:
a) Maprotiline
b) Imipramine
c) Phenelzine
d) Fluoxetine

4. Which of the following agents is related to the third-generation heterocyclic antidepressants?
a) Amitriptyline
b) Maprotiline
c) Nefazodone
d) Tranylcypromine

5. Which of the following antidepressants is a selective serotonin reuptake inhibitor?
a) Phenelzine
b) Desipramine
c) Maprotiline
d) Fluoxetine

6. Which of the following antidepressant agents is a selective inhibitor of norepinephrine reuptake?
a) Fluvoxamine
b) Maprotiline

c) Amitriptyline

d) Tranylcypromine

7. Indicate the antidepressant, which blocks the reuptake pumps for serotonin and norepinephrine:

a) Amitriptyline

b) Fluoxetine

c) Maprotiline

d) Phenelzine

8. Which of the following antidepressants is an unselective MAO blocker and produces extremely long-lasting inhibition of the enzyme?

a) Moclobemide

b) Tranylcypramine

c) Selegiline

d) Fluoxetine

9. Indicate the irreversible MAO inhibitor, which is a hydrazide derivative:

a) Moclobemide

b) Selegiline

c) Tranylcypramine

d) Phenelzine

10. Which of the following MAO inhibitors has amphetamine-like activity and is related to nonhydrazide derivatives:

a) Phenelzine

b) Moclobemide

c) Tranylcypramine

d) All of the above

11. Which of the following antidepressants is a selective short-acting MAO-A inhibitor?

a) Maprotiline

b) Amitriptyline

c) Moclobemide

d) Selegiline

12. Monoamine Oxydase A:

a) Is responsible for norepinephrine, serotonin, and tyramine metabolism

b) Is more selective for dopamine

c) Metabolizes norepinephrine and dopamine

d) Deaminates dopamine and serotonin

13. Which synapses are involved in depression?
a) Dopaminergic synapses
b) Serotoninergic synapses
c) Cholinergic synapses
d) All of the above

14. Block of which type of Monoamine Oxydase might be more selective for depression?
a) MAO-A
b) MAO-B
c) Both MAO-A and MAO-B
d) MAO-C

15. The principal mechanism of MAO inhibitor action is:
a) Blocking the amine reuptake pumps, which permits to increase the concentration of the neurotransmitter at the receptor site
b) Blocking a major degradative pathway for the amine neurotransmitters, which permits more amines to accumulate in presynaptic stores
c) Inhibition the storage of amine neurotransmitters in the vesicles of presynaptic nerve endings
d) Antagonism of alfa$_2$-norepinephrine receptors

16. The irreversible MAO inhibitors have a very high risk of developing:
a) Respiratory depression
b) Cardiovascular collapse and CNS depression
c) Hypertensive reactions to tyramine ingested in food
d) Potentially fatal agranulocytosis

17. The most dangerous pharmacodynamic interaction is between MAO inhibitors and:
a) Selective serotonin reuptake inhibitors
b) Tricyclics
c) Sympathomimetics
d) All of the above

18. Serotonin syndrome is a result of:
a) Increased stores of monoamine
b) Significant accumulation of amine neurotransmitters in the synapses
c) Both a and b
d) Depleted stores of biogenic amines

19. The therapeutic response to antidepressant drugs is usually over a period of:
a) 2-3 days
b) 2-3 weeks
c) 24 hours
d) 2-3 month

20. Which of the following antidepressants may have latency period as short as 48 hours?
a) Tranylcypromine
b) Imipramine
c) Fluoxetine
d) Amitrityline

21. Which of the following features do MAO inhibitors and tricyclic antidepressants have in common?
a) Act postsynaptically to produce their effect
b) Can precipitate hypotensive crises if certain foods are ingested
c) Increase levels of biogenic amines
d) Are useful for the manic phase of bipolar disorder

22. Tricyclic antidepressants are:
a) Highly selective serotonin reuptake inhibitors
b) Monoamine oxidase inhibitors
c) Selective norepinephrine reuptake inhibitors
d) Mixed norepinephrine and serotonin reuptake inhibitors

23. Which of the following autonomic nervous system effects is common for tricyclic antidepressants?
a) Antimuscarinic action
b) Antihistaminic action
c) Alfa adrenoreceptor-blocking action
d) All of the above

24. Indicate an effective antidepressant with minimal autonomic toxicity:
a) Amitrityline
b) Fluoxetine
c) Imipramine
d) Doxepin

25. Fluoxetine has fewer adverse effects because of:
a) Mixed norepinephrine and serotonin reuptake inhibition
b) Depleted stores of amine neurotransmitters
c) Minimal binding to cholinergic, histaminic, and alfa-adrenergic receptors
d) All of the above

26. Which of the following tricyclic and heterocyclic antidepressants has the greatest sedation?
a) Doxepin
b) Amitriptyline
c) Trazodone
d) All of the above

27. Which of the following tricyclic and heterocyclic agents has the least sedation?
a) Protriptyline
b) Trazodone
c) Amitriptyline
d) Mitrazapine

28. Indicate a tricyclic or a heterocyclic antidepressant having greatest antimuscarinic effects:
a) Desipramine
b) Amitriptyline
c) Trazodone
d) Mirtazapine

29. Indicate a tricyclic or a heterocyclic antidepressant having least antimuscarinic effects:
a) Trazodone
b) Buprorion
c) Mirtazapine
d) All of the above

30. Which of the following antidepressants has significant alfa$_2$-adrenoreceptor antagonism?
a) Amitriptyline
b) Nefazodone
c) Mirtazapine
d) Doxepin

31. Indicate the main claim for an ideal antidepressant agent:
a) A faster onset of action
b) Fewer adverse sedative and autonomic effects
c) Fewer toxicity when overdoses are taken
d) All of the above

32. Sedation, peripheral atropine-like toxicity (e.g. Cycloplegia, tachycardia, urinary retention, and constipation),orthostatic hypotension,arrhythmias, weight gain and sexual disturbances are possible adverse effects of:
a) Sertaline
b) Amitriptyline
c) Phenelsine
d) Bupropion

33. Which of the following drugs is least likely to be prescribed to patients with prostatic hypertrophy, glaucoma, coronary and cerebrovascular disease?
a) Amitriptyline
b) Paroxetine
c) Bupropion
d) Fluoxetine

34. Indicate the antidepressant agent, which is a phenyltolylpropylamine derivative:
a) Paroxetine
b) Maprotiline
c) Fluoxetine
d) Amitriptyline

35. The mechanism of fluoxetine action includes:
a) Selective inhibition of serotonine uptake in the CNS
b) Little effect on central norepinephrine or dopamine function
c) Minimal binding to cholinergic, histaminic, and alfa-adrenergic receptors
d) All of the above

36. Which of the following antidepressants is used for treatment of eating disorders, especially buliemia?
a) Amitriptyline
b) Fluoxetine
c) Imipramine
d) Tranylcypromine

37. A highly selective serotonine reuptake inhibitor is:

a) Sertaline

b) Paroxetine

c) Fluoxetine

d) All of the above

Answer Key

01-C,02-B,03-A,04C,05-D,06-B,07-A,08-B,09-D,10-C,11-C,12-A,13-B,14-A,15-B,16-C,17-D,18-C,19-B,20-A,21-C,22-D,23-D,24-B,25-C,26-D,27-A,28-B,29-D,30-C,31-D,32-B,33-A,34-C,35-D,36-B,37-D

15. Anxiolytic agents

1. Anxiolytics are used to treat:
a) Neurosis
b) Psychosis
c) Narcolepsy
d) Bipolar disorders

2. Anxiolytic agents should:
a) Relieve pain
b) Reduce anxiety and exert a calming effect
c) Improve mood and behavior in patient with psychotic symptoms
d) Produce drowsiness, encourage the onset and maintenance of a state of sleep

3. Anxiolytics are also useful for:
a) Treatment of epilepsy and seizures
b) Insomnia
c) Muscle relaxation in specific neuromuscular disorders
d) All of the above

4. Indicate the agents of choice in the treatment of most anxiety states:
a) Barbiturates
b) Benzodiazepines
c) Lithium salts
d) Phenothiazines

5. The choice of benzodiazepines for anxiety is based on:
a) A relatively high therapeutic index
b) Availability of flumazenil for treatment of overdose
c) A low risk of physiologic dependence
d) All of the above

6. Which of the following anxiolitics is a benzodiazepine derivative:
a) Buspirone
b) Clordiazepoxide
c) Meprobamate
d) Chloral hydrate

7. Indicate the benzodiazepine, which has the shortest elimination half-life:
a) Quazepam
b) Triazolam
c) Diazepam
d) Clorazepate

8. Which of the following benzodiazepines has the shortest duration of action?
a) Triazolam
b) Clorazepate
c) Prazepam
d) Clordiazepoxide

9. Which of the following benzodiazepines is less likely to cause cumulative and residual effects with multiple doses?
a) Clorazepate
b) Quazepam
c) Lorazepam
d) Prazepam

10. Anxiolytic dosage reduction is recommended:
a) In patients taking cimetidine
b) In patients with hepatic dysfunction
c) In elderly patients
d) All of the above

11. Which of the following benzodiazepines is preferred for elderly patients?
a) Clorazepate
b) Clordiazepoxide
c) Triazolam
d) Prazepam

12. Which of the following anxiolytics is preferred in patient with limited hepatic function?
a) Buspirone
b) Quazepam
c) Diazepam
d) Chlordiazepoxide

13. Indicate the mechanism of hypnotic benzodiazepine action:
a) Increasing the duration of the GABA-gated Cl⁻channel openings
b) Directly activating the chloride channels

c) Increasing the frequency of Cl⁻ channel opening events

d) All of the above

14. Which of the following anxiolytics is a partial agonist of brain 5-HT$_{1A}$receptors?

a) Buspirone

b) Alprozolam

c) Chlorazepat

d) Lorazepam

15. Indicate the competitive antagonist of BZ receptors:

a) Flumazenil

b) Buspirone

c) Picrotoxin

d) Diazepam

16. Indicate the agent, which interferes with GABA binding:

a) Chlordiazepoxide

b) Bicuculline

c) Thiopental

d) Picrotoxin

17. Antianxiety agents have:

a) Sedative and hypnotic activity

b) Muscle relaxing and anticonvulsant effects

c) Amnesic properties

d) All of the above

18. Which of the following disadvantages does not limit using benzodiazepines as antianxiety agents?

a) Tendency to develop psychologic dependence

b) A high risk of drug interactions based on liver enzyme induction

c) Synergic CNS depression with concomitant use of other drugs

d) The formation of active metabolites

19. Indicate the anxiolitic agent, which relieves anxiety without causing marked sedative effects:

a) Diazepam

b) Chlordiazepoxid

c) Buspirone

d) Clorazepate

20. Which of the following anxiolytics has minimal abuse liability?
a) Oxazepam
b) Buspirone
c) Flumazenil
d) Alprazolam

21. In contrast to benzodiazepines, buspirone:
a) Interact directly with gabaergic system
b) Has more marked hypnotic, anticonvulsant, or muscle relaxant properties
c) Causes less psychomotor impairment and does not affect driving skills
d) Has maximal abuse liability

22. Which of the following sedative-hypnotic drugs does not potentiate the CNS depressant effects of ethanol, phenothiazines, or tricyclic antidepressants?
a) Buspirone
b) Phenobarbital
c) Diazepam
d) Chloralhydrate

23. Limitation of buspirone is:
a) A low therapeutic index
b) An extremely slow onset of action
c) A high potential of development of physical dependence
d) Impairment of mentation or motor functions during working hours

24. Which drugs may be used as antianxiety agents?
a) BETA-blocking drugs
b) Clonidine - a partial agonist of alfa$_2$receptors
c) Tricyclic antidepressants
d) All of the above

25. Which of the following benzodiazepines is more likely to cause "hangover" effects such as drowsiness, dysphoria, and mental or motor depression the following day?
a) Oxazepam
b) Triazolam
c) Clorazepat
d) Lorazepam

26. Additive CNS depression can be predicted if benzodiazepines are used with:
a) Ethanol
b) Morphine
c) Clorpromazine
d) All of the above

27. Which dosage of benzodiazepines for 60-90 days may produce severe withdrawal symptoms?
a) 50-60 mg/d
b) Less than 400 mg/d
c) More than 800 mg/d
d) Less than 40 mg/d

28. Restlessness, anxiety, orthostatic hypotension, generalized seizures, severe tremor, vivid hallucination, and psychosisare possible symptoms of:
a) Tolerance
b) Withdrawal
c) Drug interactions between barbiturate and diazepam
d) None of the above

29. Flumazenil is used to:
a) Reverse the CNS depressant effects of hypnotic benzodiazepines overdose
b) Hasten recovery following use of hypnotic benzodiazepines in anesthetic and diagnostic procedure
c) Reverse benzodiazepine-induced respiratory depression
d) All of the above

30. Flumazenil given intravenously:
a) Has intermediate onset and duration of action about 2 hours
b) Acts rapidly but has a short half-life
c) Has an effect lasting 3-5 hours
d) Has duration of action longer than 6 hours

Answer Key

01-A,02-D,03-D,04-B,05-D,06-B,07-B,08-A,09-C,10-D,11-C,12-A,13-C,14-A,15-A,16-B,17-D,18-B,19-C,20-B,21-C,22-A,23-B,24-D,25-C,26-D,27-A,28-B,29-D,30-B

16. CNS stimulants

1. Agents, stimulating CNS are all of the following except:
a) Fluoxetine
b) Clozapine
c) Nootropil
d) Sydnocarb

2. Which of the following CNS stimulants are the agents of selective effect?
a) Analeptics
b) General tonics
c) Psychostimulants
d) Actoprotectors

3. Indicate CNC stimulating drugs, which are the agents of general action:
a) Nootropic agents
b) Analeptics
c) Psychostimulants
d) Antidepressants

4. Which of the following agents belongs to psychostimulants?
a) Meridil
b) Camphor
c) Piracetam
d) Pantocrin

5. Indicate the nootropic agent:
a) Sydnocarb
b) Eleuterococci extract
c) Fluoxetine
d) Piracetam

6. Which of the following agents is a respiratory analeptic?
a) Piracetam
b) Sydnocarb
c) Bemegride
d) Pantocrin

7. Indicate the CNC stimulating drug, which belongs to adaptogens:
a) Amphetamine
b) Eleuterococci extract
c) Caffeine
d) Sydnocarb

8. Actoprotectors are:
a) Stimulators, improving physical efficiency
b) Cognition enhancers, improving the highest integrative brain function
c) Stimulants, raising non-specific resistance towards stresses
d) Agents, stimulating the bulbar respiratory and vasomotor centers

9. Adaptogens cause:
a) Improvment of efficiency using physical loads and acceleration of recovery after the load
b) Stimulation of respiratory and vasomotor centers
c) Temporary relief of the feeling of tiredness, facilitating the professional work and fighting somnolence
d) Increased resistance towards stress situations and adaptation to extreme conditions

10. Indicate the CNS stimulants, which mitigate conditions of weakness or lack of tone within the entire organism or in particular organs?
a) Psychostimulants
b) Analeptics
c) General tonics
d) Antidepressants

11. Which of the following agents is a general tone-increasing drug of plant origin?
a) Meridil
b) Eleuterococci's extract
c) Pantocrin
d) Caffeine

12. Indicate a general tone-increasing drug, which is an agent of animal origin?
a) Pantocrin
b) Amphetamine
c) Sydnocarb
d) Camphor

13. Amphetamine:
a) Is a powerful stimulant of the CNS
b) Stimulates the medullar respiratory center and has an analeptic action
c) Increases motor and speech activity, mood, decreases a sense of fatigue
d) All of the above

14. The mechanism of amphetamine action is related to:
a) Direct catecholamiergic agonist action
b) Inhibition of monoamine oxydase
c) Increasing a release of catecholaminergic neurotransmitters
d) All of the above

15. Indicate the CNS stimulant, which is a piperidine derivative:
a) Meridil
b) Amphetamine
c) Caffeine
d) Sydnophen

16. Which of the following CNS psychostimulants is a sydnonymine derivative?
a) Caffeine
b) Sydnocarb
c) Meridil (methylphenidate hydrochloride)
d) Amphetamine

17. Sydnocarb causes:
a) Decreased sense of fatigue, it facilitates the professional work and fights somnolence
b) The feeling of prosperity, relaxation and euphoria
c) Influx of physical and mental forces, locomotive and speech excitation
d) Peripheral sympathomimetic action

18. Indicate the psychostimulant, which is a methylxantine derivative:
a) Caffeine
b) Sydnocarb
c) Amphetamine
d) Meridil

19. Which of the following psychostimulants acts centrally mainly by blocking adenosine receptors?
a) Meridil
b) Caffeine

c) Amphetamine

d) Sydnophen

20. Principal properties of caffeine include all of the following EXEPT:

a) Cardiac analeptic (increase the rate and the force of the cardiac contraction)

b) Adaptogenic (rise non-specific resistance towards stresses and adapt to extraordinary challenges)

c) Psychoanaleptic (decrease the feeling of tiredness, facilitates the professional work and fights somnolence)

d) Respiratory analeptic (stimulate the bulbar respiratory center)

21. Caffeine can produce all of the following effects except:

a) Coronary vasodialation

b) Relaxation of bronchial and biliary tract smooth muscles

c) Vasodialation of cerebral vessels

d) Reinforcement of the contractions and increase of the striaated muscle work

22. Caffeine does not cause:

a) Inhibition of gastric secretion

b) Hyperglycemia

c) Moderate diuretic action

d) Increase in free fatty acids

23. Therapeutic uses of caffeine include all of the following EXCEPT:

a) Cardiovascular collapse and respiratory insufficiency

b) Migraine

c) Somnolence

d) Gastric ulceration

24. Adverse effects of caffeine include all of the following EXCEPT:

a) Arrhythmias

b) Insomnia

c) Hypotension

d) Psychomotor excitation

25. Principal properties of cordiamine include all of the following EXCEPT:

a) Cardiac analeptic

b) Respiratory analeptic

c) Coronarodilatator

d) Significant abuse potential

26. Characteristics of cordiamine include all of the following EXCEPT:

a) It stimulates the CNS and facilitates the movement coordination

b) It is a respiratory analeptic of mixed action (stimulates both the medullar respiratory center and chemoreceptor of carotid sinus zone)

c) It decreases the aortic and coronary flow

d) It counteracts the central depression produced by other drugs (barbiturates)

27. Cordiamine is useful in the treatment of:

a) Hypotension

b) Coronary insufficiency

c) Respiratory insufficiency

d) All of the above

28. Respiratory and cardiac analeptics are all of the following agents EXCEPT:

a) Cordiamine

b) Bemegride

c) Caffeine

d) Camphor

29. Bemegride:

a) Stimulates the medullar respiratory center (central effect)

b) Stimulates hemoreceptors of carotid sinus zone (reflector action)

c) Is a mixed agent (both central and reflector effects)

d) Is a spinal analeptic

30. Which of the following CNS stimulants belongs to nootropics?

a) Camphor

b) Pantocrin

c) Sydnocarb

d) Piracetam

31. Characteristics of nootropics include all of the following EXCEPT:

a) Selective influence on the brain

b) Improvement the ability to communicate with peers

c) Decline in the highest integrative brain functions

d) Increase in energetic exchange of the brain cells

32. Which of the following statements concerning nootropics is not correct?

a) They improve the highest integrative brain functions (memory, learning, understanding, thinking and the capacity for concentration)

b) They stimulate the bulbar respiratory center

c) They stimulate existing neuronal synapses to optimum performance (adaptive capacity)

d) They stimulate existing neuronal synapses to damaging influences, such as disturbances of the energy and neurotransmitter metabolism or ischemia (protective capacity)

33. Features of piracetam include all of the following EXCEPT:
a) It is a GABA derivative
b) It does not influence the neuro-vegetative function
c) Improvement begins in the 3'rd week
d) It has a high potential of toxicity

34. Piracetam can produce all of the following effects EXCEPT:
a) Antipsychotic
b) Anticonvulsant
c) Psychometabolic
d) Antihypoxic

35. Piracetam is widely used for the treatment of:
a) Senile dementia
b) Asthenia
c) Chronic alcoholism
d) All of the above

36. Indicate the CNS stimulant, which is used in pediatric medicine, as it improves the communication with the child,increases the ability to study and communication with peers, improves school-performance?
a) Meridil
b) Piracetam
c) Bemegride
d) Amphetamine

37. Which of the following CNS stimulants is used for the cerebral stroke treatment?
a) Pantocrin
b) Sydnocarb
c) Piracetam
d) Caffeine

Answer Key

01-B,02-C,03-B,04-A,05-D,06-C,07-B,08-A,09-D,10-C,11-B,12-A,13-D,14-D,15-A,16-B,17-A,18-A,19-B,20-B,21-C,22-A,23-D,24-C,25-D,26-C,27-D,28-B,29-A,30-D,31-C,32-B,33-D,34-A,35-D,36-B,37-C

17. Drugs of abuse

1. Psychologic dependence is:
a) Decreased responsiveness to a drug following repeated exposure
b) A combination of certain drug-specific symptoms that occur on sudden discontinuation of a drug
c) Compulsive drug-seeking behavior
d) All of the above

2. Tolerance is associated with:
a) An ability to compensate for the drug effect
b) Increased disposition of the drug after chronic use
c) Compensatory changes in receptors, effector enzymes, or membrane actions of the drug
d) All of the above

3. Addiction is associated with the existence of:
a) Psychological dependence
b) Physiological dependence
c) Tolerance
d) All of the above

4. Substances causing narco- and glue sniffings are all of the following EXCEPT:
a) Stimulants
b) Antipsychotic drugs
c) Psychedelics
d) Sedative drugs

5. Which of the following abused drugs do not belong to sedative agents?
a) Barbiturates
b) Tranquilizers
c) Cannabinoids
d) Opioids

6. Psychedelics are all of following agents EXCEPT:
a) Cocaine
b) LSD
c) Marijuana
d) Volatile substances (glues, solvents, volatile nitrites and nitrous oxide)

7. In contrast to morphine, heroin is:
a) Used clinically
b) More addictive and fast-acting
c) More effective orally
d) Less potent and long-acting

8. The acute course of opioid withdrawal may last:
a) 3-4 days
b) 7-10 days
c) 3-4 weeks
d) 26-30 weeks

9. Indicate the sedative-hypnotic agent, which has the highest abuse potential:
a) Buspirone
b) Diazepam
c) Phenobarbital
d) Zolpidem

10. Characteristics of barbiturate intoxication (2-3 dose) include all of the following EXCEPT:
a) Pleasant feelings of the "blow" in the head, vertigo, myasthenia, stupor
b) Perceptual distortion of surroundings, disorders of thinking, behavior
c) Locomotive, speech excitation, sharp swings from a cheerful mood to an aggressive state
d) Sleep with the subsequent weakness and headaches

11. Barbiturate abstinent syndrome is shown by:
a) Crisis by 3 day of abstention
b) Anxiety, mydriasis, myasthenia, muscular convulsions, vomiting, diarrhea
c) Psychosis as delirium (color visual and auditory hallucinations)
d) All of the above

12. Which one of the following tranquilizers belongs to strong euphorizing agents?
a) Mebicarum
b) Buspirone
c) Diazepam
d) Chlordiazepoxide

13. Tranquilizers intoxication (5-10 tablets) features include:
a) Euphoria, burst of energy, increase in motor activity, wave warmth all over the body
b) Visual hallucinations, a distorted feelling of time and space
c) Physical bliss, body lightness, a wish to fly, motionlessness
d) Synaesthesia (the sounds can be tensed, the colors can be heard)

14. Which of the following abused drugs is related to stimulants?
a) Cocaine
b) Amphetamine
c) Caffeine
d) All of the above

15. Cocaine exerts its central action by:
a) Inhibiting phosphodiesterase
b) Increasing a release of catecholaminergic neurotransmitters, including dopamine
c) Inhibiting dopamine and norepinephrine reuptake
d) Altering serotonin turnover

16. "Crack" is a derivative of:
a) Opium
b) LSD
c) Cocaine
d) Cannabis

17. Cocaine intoxication appears by:
a) Short clouding of consciousness, lightness of body and a feeling of flight
b) Wave warmth all over the body, physical bliss, motionlessness
c) Clear consciousness, improved mood, influx of physical and spiritual forces, locomotive and speech excitation, reappraisal of personality
d) All of the above

18. Which of the following stimulants is related to psychedelics?
a) "ecstasy" (methylenedioxymethamphetamine)
b) Cocaine
c) "crack" (cocaine free base)
d) Caffeine

19. Cocaine may cause:
a) Powerful vasoconstrictive reactions resulting in myocardial infarctions
b) The multiple brain perfusion defects

c) Spontaneous abortion during pregnancy

d) All of the above

20. Characteristics of cocaine abstinent syndrome include all of the following phases EXCEPT:

a) Feeling of depression, irritability, confusion, insomnia (the first 3 days)

b) Depression, apathy, excessive appetite, a wish to sleep (the subsequent 1-2 days)

c) Psychosis as color visual and auditory hallucinations (for 3 day)

d) New attack of depression, anxiety, irritability, dullness, intense thirst for cocaine (after 1-5 days improvement)

21. Overdoses of cocaine are usually rapidly fatal from:

a) Respiratory depression

b) Arrhythmias

c) Seizures

d) All of the above

22. Which of the following agents is related to hallucinogens?

a) Heroin

b) LSD

c) Cocaine

d) Opium

23. LSD produces:

a) Mood swings

b) Impaired memory, difficulty in thinking, poor judgment

c) Perceptual distortion

d) All of the above

24. LSD decreases in brain:

a) $5\text{-}HT_2$ receptor densities

b) $GABA_A$-benzodiazepine receptor densities

c) Adrenergic receptor densities

d) D_2 receptor densities

25. Which of the following agents is related to cannabis?

a) Heroin

b) Ecstasy

c) Hashish

d) Crack

26. The early stage of cannabis intoxication is characterized by:
a) Euphoria, uncontrolled laugher
b) Alteration of time sense, depersonalization
c) Sharpened vision
d) All of the above

27. Which of the following physiologic signs is a characteristic of cannabis intoxication?
a) Bradycardia
b) Reddening of the conjunctiva
c) Miosis
d) Nausea and vomiting

28. Industrial solvent inhalation causes:
a) Quick intoxication, lasting only 5-15 minutes
b) Euphoria, relaxed "drunk" feeling
c) Disorientation, slow passage of time and possible hallucinations
d) All of the above

29. Indicate the drugs of choice for reversing the withdrawal syndrome:
a) Benzodiazepines
b) Neuroleptics
c) Antidepressants
d) All of the above

Answer Key

01-C,02-D,03-D,04-B,05-C,06-A,07-B,08-B,09-C,10-B,11-D,12-C,13-A,14-D,15-C,16-C,17-D,18-A,19-D,20-C,21-D,22-B,23-D,24-A,25-C,26-D,27-B,28-D,29-D

18. General anesthetics

1. The state of "general anesthesia" usually includes:
a) Analgesia
b) Loss of consciousness, inhibition of sensory and autonomic reflexes
c) Amnesia
d) All of the above

2. Inhaled anesthetics and intravenous agents having general anesthetic properties:
a) Directly activate $GABA_A$ receptors
b) Facilitate GABA action but have no direct action on $GABA_A$ receptors
c) Reduce the excitatory glutamatergic neurotransmission
d) Increase the duration of opening of nicotine-activated potassium channels

3. Indicate the anesthetic, which is an inhibitor of NMDA glutamate receptors:
a) Thiopental
b) Halothane
c) Ketamine
d) Sevoflurane

4. An ideal anesthetic drug would:
a) Induces anesthesia smoothly and rapidly and secure rapid recovery
b) Posses a wide margin of safety
c) Be devoid of adverse effects
d) All of the above

5. Which of the following general anesthetics belongs to inhalants?
a) Thiopental
b) Desfluran
c) Ketamine
d) Propofol

6. Indicate the anesthetic, which is used intravenously:
a) Propofol
b) Halothane
c) Desflurane
d) Nitrous oxide

7. Which of the following inhalants is a gas anesthetic?
a) Halothane
b) Isoflurane
c) Nitrous oxide
d) Desflurane

8. Sevoflurane has largely replaced halothane and isoflurane as an inhalation anesthetic of choice because:
a) Induction of anesthesia is achieved more rapidly and smoothly
b) Recovery is more rapid
c) It has low post- anesthetic organ toxicity
d) All of the above

9. The limitation of sevoflurane is:
a) High incidence of coughing and laryngospasm
b) Chemically unstable
c) Centrally mediated sympathetic activation leading to a rise of BP and HR
d) Hepatotoxicity

10. Which of the following inhalants lacks sufficient potency to produce surgical anesthesia by itself and therefore is commonly used with another or inhaled intravenous anesthetic?
a) Halothane
b) Sevofluranc
c) Nitrous oxide
d) Desflurane

11. Which of the following inhaled anesthetics has rapid onset and recovery?
a) Nitrous oxide
b) Desflurane
c) Sevoflurane
d) All of the above

12. Indicate the inhaled anesthetic, which reduces arterial pressure and heart rate:
a) Isoflurane
b) Halothane
c) Desflurane
d) Nitrous oxide

13. Which of the following inhaled anesthetics causes centrally mediated sympathetic activation leading to a rise in blood pressure and heart rate?
a) Desflurane
b) Sevoflurane
c) Nitrous oxide
d) Isofurane

14. Indicated the inhaled anesthetic, which decreases the ventilatory response to hypoxia:
a) Sevoflurane
b) Nitrous oxide
c) Desflurane
d) Halothane

15. Which of the following inhaled anesthetics is an induction agent of choice in patient with airway problems?
a) Desfurane
b) Nitrous oxide
c) Halothane
 d) None of the above

16. Indicate the inhaled anesthetic, which causes the airway irritation:
a) Nitrous oxide
b) Sevoflurane
c) Halothane
d) Desflurane

17. Which of the following inhaled anesthetics increases cerebral blood flow least of all?
a) Sevoflurane
b) Nitrous oxide
c) Isoflurane
d) Desflurane

18. Indicate the inhaled anesthetic, which should be avoided in patients with a history of seizure disorders:
a) Enflurane
b) Nitrous oxide
c) Sevoflurane
d) Desflurane

19. Which of the following inhaled anesthetics can produce hepatic necrosis?
a) Soveflurane
b) Desflurane
c) Halothane
d) Nitrous oxide

20. Indicated the inhaled anesthetic, which may cause nephrotoxicity:
a) Halothane
b) Soveflurane
c) Nitrous oxide
d) Diethyl ether

21. Which of the following inhaled anesthetics decreases metheonine synthase activity and causes megaloblastic anemia?
a) Desflurane
b) Halothane
c) Nitrous oxide
d) Soveflurane

22. Unlike inhaled anesthetics, intravenous agents such as thiopental, etomidate, and propofol:
a) Have a faster onset and rate of recovery
b) Provide a state of conscious sedation
c) Are commonly used for induction of anesthesia
d) All of the above

23. Indicate the intravenous anesthetic, which is an ultra-short-acting barbiturate:
a) Fentanyl
b) Thiopental
c) Midazolam
d) Ketamine

24. Indicate the intravenous anesthetic, which is a benzodiazepine derivative:
a) Midazolam
b) Thiopental
c) Ketamin
d) Propofol

25. Which of the following agents is used to accelerate recovery from the sedative actions of intravenous benzodiazepines?
a) Naloxone
b) Flumazenil
c) Ketamine
d) Fomepizole

26. Neuroleptanalgesia has all of the following properties EXCEPT:
a) Droperidol and fentanyl are commonly used
b) It can be used with nitrous oxide to provide neuroleptanesthesia
c) Hypertension is a common consequence
d) Confusion and mental depression can occur as adverse effects

27. Which of the following intravenous anesthetics has antiemetic actions?
a) Thiopental
b) Propofol
c) Ketamine
d) Fentanyl

28. Indicate the intravenous anesthetic, which causes minimal cardiovascular and respiratory depressant effects:
a) Propofol
b) Thiopental
c) Etomidate
d) Midazolam

29. Indicate the intravenous anesthetic, which produces dissociative anesthesia:
a) Midazolam
b) Ketamine
c) Fentanyl
d) Thiopental

30. Ketamine anesthesia is associated with:
a) Cardiovascular stimulation
b) Increased cerebral blood flow, oxygen consumption and intracranial pressure
c) Disorientation, sensory and perceptual illusions, and vivid dreams following anesthesia
d) All of the above

Answer Key

01-D,02-A,03-C,04-D,05-B,06-A,07-C,08-D,09-B,10-C,11-D,12-B,13-A,14-B,15-C,16-D,17-B,18-A,19-C,20-B,21-C,22-D,23-B,24-A,25-B,26-C,27-B,28-C,29-B,30-D

19. Drugs acting on respiratory system

1. Following drugs directly activate the respiratory center EXCEPT:
a) Bemegride
b) Caffeine
c) Aethymizole
d) Cytiton

2. The mechanism of Cytiton action is:
a) Direct activation of the respiratory center
b) The reflex mechanism
c) The mixed mechanism
d) None of the above

3. Indicate the drug belonging to antitussives of narcotic type of action:
a) Glaucine hydrochloride
b) Aethylmorphine hydrochloride
c) Tusuprex
d) Libexine

4. Tick out the drug belonging to non-narcotic antitussives:
a) Libexine
b) Tusuprex
c) Codeine
d) Aethylmorphine hydrochloride

5. Indicate the expectorant with the reflex mechanism:
a) Sodium benzoate
b) Derivatives of Ipecacucnha and Thermopsis
c) Trypsin
d) Ambroxol

6. Tick the antitussive agent with a peripheral effect:
a) Codeine
b) Tusuprex
c) Libexine
d) Glaucine hydrochloride

7. All of these drugs contain free sulfhydryl groups EXCEPT:
a) Acetylcysteine
b) Ambroxol
c) Bromhexin
d) Trypsin

8. Which of the following drugs is proteolytic enzyme?
a) Potassium iodide
b) Desoxiribonuclease
c) Carbocysteine
d) Acetylcysteine

9. All of the following drugs destroy disulfide bonds of proteoglycans, which causes depolymerization and reduction of viscosity of sputum, EXCEPT:
a) Acetylcysteine
b) Ambroxol
c) Desoxiribonuclease
d) Bromhexin

10. Which of these groups of drugs is used for asthma treatment?
a) Methylxanthines
b) M-cholinoblocking agents
c) Beta$_2$- stimulants
d) All of above

11. Tick the drug belonging to non-selective beta$_2$-adrenomimics:
a) Salbutamol
b) Isoprenaline
c) Salmeterol
d) Terbutaline

12. Select the side-effect characteristic for non-selective beta$_2$-adrenomimics:
a) Depression of the breathing centre
b) Tachycardia
c) Peripheral vasoconstriction
d) Dry mouth

13. Pick out the bronchodilator drug related to xanthine:
a) Atropine
b) Orciprenaline
c) Adrenaline
d) Theophylline

14. Pick out the bronchodilator drug belonging to sympathomimics:
a) Isoprenaline
b) Ephedrine
c) Atropine
d) Salbutamol

15. The mechanism of methylxanthines action is:
a) Inhibition of the enzyme phosphodiesterase
b) Beta$_2$-adrenoreceptor stimulation
c) Inhibition of the production of inflammatory cytokines
d) Inhibition of M-cholinoreceptors

16. Which of the following M-cholinoblocking agents is used especially as an anti-asthmatic?
a) Atropine
b) Ipratropium
c) Platiphylline
d) Metacin

17. Indicate the side effect of Theophylline:
a) Bradycardia
b) Increased myocardial demands for oxygen
c) Depression of respiratory centre
d) Elevation of the arterial blood pressure

18. All of the following drugs are inhaled glucocorticoids EXCEPT:
a) Triamcinolone
b) Beclometazone
c) Sodium cromoglycate
d) Budesonide

19. Choose the drug belonging to membranestabilizing agents:
a) Zileutin
b) Sodium cromoglycate
c) Zafirlucast
d) Montelucast

20. Tick the drug which is a 5-lipoxygenase inhibitor:
a) Budesonide
b) Sodium cromoglycate
c) Zileutin
d) Beclometazone

21. Indicate the drug which is a leucotriene receptor antagonist:
a) Sodium cromoglycate
b) Zafirlucast
c) Zileutin
d) Triamcinolone

Answer key

01-D,02-B,03-B,04-B,05-B,06-C,07-D,08-B,09-C,10-D,11-B,12-B,13-D,14-B
15-A,16-B,17-B,18-C,19-B,20-C,21-B

20. Drugs used in gastrointestinal diseases

1. Tick the main approach of peptic ulcer treatment:
a) Neutralization of gastric acid
b) Eradication of Helicobacter pylori
c) Inhibition of gastric acid secretion
d) All the above

2. Gastric acid secretion is under the control of the following agents EXCEPT:
a) Histamine
b) Acetylcholine
c) Serotonin
d) Gastrin

3. Indicate the drug belonging to proton pump inhibitors:
a) Pirenzepine
b) Ranitidine
c) Omeprazole
d) Trimethaphan

4. All of the following agents intensify the secretion of gastric glands EXCEPT:
a) Pepsin
b) Gastrin
c) Histamine
d) Carbonate mineral waters

5. Which of the following drugs is an agent of substitution therapy?
a) Gastrin
b) Hydrochloric acid
c) Hystamine
d) Carbonate mineral waters

6. Choose the drug which is a H2-receptor antagonist:
a) Omeprazole
b) Pirenzepine
c) Carbenoxolone
d) Ranitidine

7. All of the following drugs are proton pump inhibitors EXCEPT:
a) Pantoprozole
b) Omeprazole
c) Famotidine
d) Rabeprazole

8. Indicate the drug belonging to M1-cholinoblockers:
a) Cimetidine
b) Ranitidine
c) Pirenzepin
d) Omeprazole

9. Which of the following drugs may cause reversible gynecomastia?

a) Omeprazole
b) Pirenzepine
c) Cimetidine
d) Sucralfate

10. Tick the drug forming a physical barrier to HCL and Pepsin:
a) Ranitidine
b) Sucralfate
c) Omeprazole
d) Pirenzepine

11. Which drug is an analog of prostaglandin E_1?
a) Misoprostole
b) De-nol
c) Sucralfate
d) Omeprazole

12. Select the drug stimulating the protective function of the mucous barrier and the stability of the mucous membrane against damaging factors:
a) De-nol
b) Sucralfate
c) Misoprostol
d) Omeprazole

13. Most of drugs are antacids EXCEPT:
a) Misoprostol
b) Maalox

c) Mylanta
d) Almagel

14. Indicate the drug that cause metabolic alkalosis:
a) Sodium bicarbonate
b) Cimetidine
c) Pepto-Bismol
d) Carbenoxolone

15. Choose the drug that causes constipation:
a) Sodium bicarbonate
b) Aluminium hydroxide
c) Calcium carbonate
d) Magnesium oxide

16. All of the following drugs stimulate appetite EXCEPT:
a) Vitamins
b) Bitters
c) Fepranone
d) Insulin

17. Select an anorexigenic agent affecting serotoninergic system:
a) Fenfluramine
b) Fepranone
c) Desopimone
d) Masindole

18. All of the following drugs intensify gastrointestinal motility EXCEPT:
a) Papaverine
b) Metoclopramide
c) Domperidone
d) Cisapride

19. Choose an emetic drug of central action:
a) Ipecacuanha derivatives
b) Promethazine
c) Tropisetron
d) Apomorphine hydrochloride

20.Tick the mechanism of Metoclopramide antiemetic action:
a) $H_1$and H_2-receptor blocking effect
b) M-cholinoreceptor stimulating effect

c) D $_2$ -dopamine and 5-HT $_3$ -serotonin receptor blocking effect

d) M-cholinoblocking effect

21. Select the emetic agent having a reflex action:

a) Ipecacuanha derivatives

b) Apomorphine hydroclorid

c) Chlorpromazine

d) Metoclopramide

22. All of the following drugs are antiemetics EXCEPT:

a) Metoclopramide

b) Ondansetron

c) Chlorpromazine

d) Apomorphine hydrochloride

23. Indicate an antiemetic agent which is related to neuroleptics:

a) Metoclopramide

b) Nabilone

c) Tropisetron

d) Prochlorperazine

24. All of these drugs reduce intestinal peristalsis EXCEPT:

a) Loperamide

b) Cisapride

c) Methyl cellulose

d) Magnesium aluminium silicate

25. Indicate the laxative drug belonging to osmotic laxatives:

a) Docusate sodium

b) Bisacodyl

c) Phenolphthalein

d) Sodium phosphate

26. The mechanism of stimulant purgatives is:

a) Increasing the volume of non-absorbable solid residue

b) Increasing motility and secretion

c) Altering the consistency of the feces

d) Increasing the water content

27. Choose the drug irritating the gut and causing increased peristalsis:

a) Phenolphthalein

b) Methyl cellulose

c) Proserine
d) Mineral oil

28. All of the following drugs stimulate bile production and bile secretion EXCEPT:
a) Chenodiol
b) Cholenszyme
c) Oxaphenamide
d) Cholosas

29. Tick the stimulant of bile production of vegetable origin:
a) Oxaphenamide
b) Papaverine
c) Cholenzyme
d) Cholosas

30. Select the drug which inhibits peristalsis:
a) Castor oil
b) Bisacodyl
c) Loperamide
d) Sorbitol

Answer Key

01-D,02-C,03-C,04-A,05-B,07-C,08-C,09-C,10-B,11-A,12-C,13-A,14-A,15-B,16-C,17-A,18-A,19-D,20-C,21-A,22-D,23-D,24-B,25-D,26-B,27-A,28-A,29-D,30-C

21. Drugs acting on hematopoietic system

1. Following drugs stimulate erythrogenesis EXCEPT:
a) Iron dextran
b) Vitamine B_{12}
c) Methotrexate
d) Folic acid

2. Choose the drug depressing erythrogenesis:
a) Radioactive phosphorus 32
b) Ferrous sulfate
c) Molgramostim
d) Folic acid

3. Which drug does not influence leucopoiesis?
a) Filgrastim
b) Erythropoetin
c) Doxorubicin
d) Methotrexate

4. All of the following drugs used for iron deficiency anemia EXCEPT:
a) Ferrous sulfate
b) Folic acid
c) Ferrous gluconate
d) Ferrous fumarate

5. Tick the drug for parenteral iron therapy:
a) Ferrous sulfate
b) Fercoven
c) Ferrous lactate
d) Ferrous fumarate

6. Indicate the drug which increases absorption of iron from intestine:
a) Cyanocobalamin
b) Folic acid
c) Ascorbic acid
d) Erythropoetin

7. The drugs used for oral administration EXCLUDE:
a) Ferrous sulfate
b) Fercoven
c) Ferrous lactate
d) Ferrous fumarate

8. Pernicious anemia is developed due to deficiency of:
a) Erythropoetin
b) Vitamin B $_{12}$
c) Iron
d) Vitamin B$_6$

9. Select the drug used for pernicious anemia:
a) Ferrous lactate
b) Cyanocobalamin
c) Iron dextran
d) Ferrous gluconate

10. An adverse effect of oral iron therapy is:
a) Anemia
b) Thrombocytopenia
c) Headache
d) Constipation

11. Choose the drug which contains cobalt atom:
a) Folic acid
b) Iron dextran
c) Cyanocobalamine
d) Ferrous gluconate

12. Tick the drug used in aplastic anemia:
a) Fercoven
b) Cyanocobalamine
c) Epoetin alpha
d) Folic acid

13. Select the drug of granulocyte colony-stimulating factor:
a) Filgrastim
b) Methotrexate
c) Erythropoetin
d) Doxorubicin

Answer Key

01-C,02-A,03-B,04-B,05-B ,06-C,07-B,08-B,09-B,10-D,11-C,12-C,13-A

22. Drugs used in disorders of coagulation

1. All of the following physiologic reactions are involved in the control of bleeding EXCEPT:
a) Platelet adhesion reaction
b) Platelet release reaction
c) Activation of the antifibrinolytic system
d) Triggering of the coagulation process

2. Which of the following substances is synthesized within vessel walls and inhibits thrombogenesis?
a) Thromboxane A_2 (TXA$_2$)
b) Prostacyclin (PGI $_2$)
c) Prostaglandin ((PGE)
d) None of the above

3. All of the following groups of drugs are for thrombosis treatment EXCEPT:
a) Anticoagulant drugs
b) Antifibrinolitic drugs
c) Fibrinolitic drugs
d) Antiplatelet drugs

4. Pick out the drug belonging to anticoagulants of direct action:
a) Aspirin
b) Heparin
c) Dicumarol
d) Phenprocoumon

5. Which of the following drugs has low-molecular weight?
a) Dicumarol
b) Enoxaparin
c) Phenprocoumon
d) Heparin

6. Indicate the drug belonging to antagonists of heparin:
a) Aspirin
b) Dicumarol
c) Dalteparin
d) Protamine sulfate

7. Tick the drug used as an oral anticoagulant:
a) Heparin
b) Daltreparin
c) Dicumarol
d) Enoxaparin

8. All of the following drugs are indirect acting anticoagulants EXCEPT:
a) Dicumarol
b) Warfarin
c) Dalteparin
d) Phenindione

9. Which of the following drugs belongs to coumarin derivatives?
a) Heparin
b) Enoxaparin
c) Dalteparin
d) Warfarin

10. All of these drugs are antiplatelet agents EXCEPT:
a) Aspirin
b) Urokinase
c) Ticlopidine
d) Clopidogrel

11. Mechanism of aspirin action is:
a) Converts inactive plasminogen into active plasmin
b) Inhibits COX and thus thromboxane synthesis
c) Enhances the interaction between antitrombin III and both thrombin and the factors involved in the intrinsic clotting cascade
d) Inhibits the glycoprotein IIb/IIIa complex

12. Which of the following drugs is an inhibitor of platelet glycoprotein IIb/ IIIa receptors?
a) Aspirin
b) Clopidogrel
c) Ticlopidine
d) Abciximab

13. Which of the following drugs is fiibrinolytic?
a) Ticlopidine
b) Streptokinase
c) Aspirin
d) Warfarin

14. Fibrinolytic drugs are used for following EXCEPT:
a) Central deep venous thrombosis
b) Multiple pulmonary emboli
c) Heart failure
d) Acute myocardial infarction

15. Indicate the drug belonging to fibrinoliytic inhibitors:
a) Aminocapronic acid
b) Ticlopidine
c) Streptokinase
d) Vitamin K

16. Aminocapronic acid is a drug of choice for treatment of:
a) Acute myocardial infarction
b) Bleeding from fibrinolytic therapy
c) Heart failure
d) Multiple pulmonary emboli

Answer Key

01-C,02-B,03-B,04-B,05-B,06-D,07-C,08-C,09-D,10-B,11-B,12-D,13-B,14-C,15-A,16-A

23. Drugs used for treatment of heart failure

1. All of the following are normally involved in the pathogenesis of heart failure EXCEPT:
a) A cardiac lesion that impairs cardiac output
b) An increase in peripheral vascular resistance
c) A decrease in preload
d) An increase in sodium and water retention

2. All of the following are compensatory mechanisms that occur during the pathogenesis of congestive heart failure EXCEPT:
a) An increase in ventricular end-diastolic volume
b) An increase in the concentration of plasma catecholamines
c) An increase in vagal tone
d) Increased activity of the renin-angiotensin-aldosterone system

3. All of the following are recommended at the initial stages of treating patients with heart failure EXCEPT:
a) Reduced salt intake
b) Verapamil
c) ACE inhibitors
d) Diuretics

4. All of the following agents belong to cardiac glycosides EXCEPT:
a) Digoxin
b) Strophantin K
c) Amrinone
d) Digitoxin

5. The non-glycoside positive inotropic drug is:
a) Digoxin
b) Strophantin K
c) Dobutamine
d) Digitoxin

6. Sugar molecules in the structure of glycosides influence:
a) Cardiotonic action
b) Pharmacokinetic properties

c) Toxic properties
d) All of the above

7. Aglycone is essential for:
a) Plasma protein binding
b) Half-life
c) Cardiotonic action
d) Metabolism

8. Choose the derivative of the plant Foxglove (Digitalis):
a) Digoxin
b) Strophantin K
c) Dobutamine
d) Amrinone

9. All of the following statements regarding cardiac glycosides are true EXCEPT:
a) They inhibit the activity of the Na+/K+-ATPase
b) They decrease intracellular concentrations of calcium in myocytes
c) They increase vagal tone
d) They have a very low therapeutic index

10. All of the following statements regarding cardiac glycosides are true EXCEPT:
a) Digoxin is a mild inotrope
b) Digoxin increases vagal tone
c) Digoxin has a longer half-life than digitoxin
d) Digoxin acts by inhibiting the Na+/K+ ATPase

11. The most cardiac manifestation of glycosides intoxication is:
a) Atrioventricular junctional rhythm
b) Second-degree atrioventricular blockade
c) Ventricular tachycardia
d) All the above

12. The manifestations of glycosides intoxication are:
a) Visual changes
b) Ventricular tachyarrhythmias
c) Gastrointestinal disturbances
d) All the above

13. For digitalis-induced arrhythmias the following drug is favored:
a) Verapamil
b) Amiodarone
c) Lidocaine
d) Propanolol

14. In very severe digitalis intoxication the best choice is to use:
a) Lidocaine
b) Digibind (Digoxin immune fab)
c) Oral potassium supplementation
d) Reducing the dose of the drug

15. All of the following statements regarding cardiac glycoside-induced ventricular tachyarrhythmias are true EXCEPT:
a) Lidocaine is a drug of choice in treatment
b) Digibind should be used in life-threatening cases
c) They occur more frequently in patients with hyperkalemia than in those with hypokalemia
d) They are more likely to occur in patients with a severely damaged heart

16. This drug is a selective beta-1 agonist:
a) Digoxin
b) Dobutamine
c) Amrinone
d) Dopamine

17. Tolerance to this inotropic drug develops after a few days:
a) Amrinone
b) Amiodarone
c) Dobutamine
d) Adenosine

18. This drug inhibits breakdown of cAMP in vascular smooth muscle:
a) Digoxin
b) Dobutamine
c) Amrinone
d) Dopamine

19. This drug is useful for treating heart failure because it increases the inotropic state and reduces afterload:
a) Amiodarone
b) Amrinone
c) Propanolol
d) Enalapril

20. This drug acts by inhibiting type III cyclic nucleotide phosphodiesterase:
a) Amiodarone
b) Milrinone
c) Propanolol
d) Enalapril

21. All of the following statements regarding inhibitors of type III phosphodiesterase are true EXCEPT:
a) They raise cAMP concentrations in cardiac myocytes
b) They reduce afterload
c) They show significant cross-tolerance with beta-receptor agonists
d) They are associated with a significant risk for cardiac arrhythmias

22. All of the following drugs are used in the treatment of severe congestive heart failure EXCEPT:
a) Verapamil
b) Digoxin
c) Dobutamine
d) Dopamine

23. Drugs most commonly used in chronic heart failure are:
a) Cardiac glycosides
b) Diuretics
c) Angiotensin-converting enzyme inhibitors
d) All the above

24. All of the following statements concerning angiotensin converting enzyme (ACE) inhibitors are true EXCEPT:
a) They act by inhibiting the ability of renin to convert angiotensinogen to angiotensin I.
b) Enalapril is a prodrug that is converted to an active metabolite
c) They reduce secretion of aldosterone
d) They can produce hyperkalemia in combination with a potassium-sparing diuretic

25. All of the following effects of ACE inhibitors may be useful in treating heart failure EXCEPT:
a) They decrease afterload
b) They increase circulating catecholamine levels
c) They reduce reactive myocardial hypertrophy
d) They increase myocardial beta-1 adrenergic receptor density

26. All of the following statements concerning the use of angiotensin-converting enzyme (ACE) inhibitors in the treatment of heart failure are true EXCEPT:
a) They improve hemodynamics by decreasing afterload
b) They can increase plasma cholesterol levels
c) They may slow the progression of heart failure by preventing myocardial and vascular remodeling
d) They are effective first-line agents in the treatment of chronic heart failure

Answer Key

01-C,02-C,03-B,04-C,05-C,06-B,07-C,08-A,09-B,10-C,11-D,12-D,13-C,14-B,
15-C,16-B,17-C,18-C,19-B,20-B,21-C,22-A,23-D,24-A,25-B,26-B

24. Antiarrhythmic agents

1. This drug is a Class IA antiarrhythmic drug:
a) Sotalol
b) Propranolol
c) Verapamil
d) Quinidine

2. This drug is a Class IC antiarrhythmic drug:
a) Flecainide
b) Sotalol
c) Lidocaine
d) Verapamil

3. This drug is a Class IC antiarrhythmic drug:
a) Flecainide
b) Sotalol
c) Lidocaine
d) Verapamil

4. This drug is a Class II antiarrhythmic drug:
a) Flecainide
b) Propranolol
c) Lidocaine
d) Verapamil

5. This drug is a Class III antiarrhythmic drug:
a) Flecainide
b) Sotalol
c) Lidocaine
d) Verapamil

6. This drug prolongs repolarization:
a) Flecainide
b) Sotalol
c) Lidocaine
d) Verapamil

7. This drug is a Class IV antiarrhythmic drug:
a) Flecainide
b) Sotalol
c) Lidocaine
d) Verapamil

8. This drug is used in treating supraventricular tachycardias:
a) Digoxin
b) Dobutamine
c) Amrinone
d) Dopamine

9. This drug is associated with Torsades de pointes.
a) Flecainide
b) Sotalol
c) Lidocaine
d) Verapamil

10. This drug has beta-adrenergic blocking activity :
a) Flecainide
b) Sotalol
c) Lidocaine
d) Verapamil

11. This drug is useful in terminating atrial but not ventricular tachycardias:
a) Flecainide
b) Sotalol
c) Lidocaine
d) Verapamil

12. This is a drug of choice for acute treatment of ventricular tachycardias:
a) Flecainide
b) Sotalol
c) Lidocaine
d) Verapamil

13. This drug is contraindicated in patients with moderate to severe heart failure:
a) Nifedipine
b) Verapamil
c) Both of the above
d) None of the above

14. This drug is an effective bronchodilator:
a) Nifedipine
b) Verapamil
c) Both of the above.
d) None of the above

15. This drug is used intravenously to terminate supraventricular tachycardias:
a) Nifedipine
b) Verapamil
c) Both of the above
d) None of the above

16. This drug has a little or no direct effect on chronotropy and dromotropy at normal doses
a) Nifedipine
b) Diltiazem
c) Verapamil
d) All of the above

17. This drug acts by inhibiting slow calcium channels in the SA and AV nodes:
a) Quinidine
b) Adenosine
c) Flecainide
d) Diltiazem

18. All of the following statements regarding verapamil are true EXCEPT:
a) It blocks L-type calcium channels
b) It increases heart rate
c) It relaxes coronary artery smooth muscle
d) It depresses cardiac contractility

19. All of the following calcium channel blockers are useful in the treatment of cardiac arrhythmias EXCEPT:
a) Bepridil
b) Diltiazem
c) Verapamil
d) Nifedipine

20. All of the following are common adverse effects of calcium channel blockers EXCEPT:

a) Skeletal muscle weakness

b) Dizziness

c) Headache

d) Flushing

21. Tick the adverse reactions characteristic for lidocaine:

a) Agranulocytosis, leucopenia

b) Extrapyramidal disorders

c) Hypotension, paresthesias, convulsions

d) Bronchospasm, dyspepsia

Answer Key

01-D,02-C,03-A,04-B,05-B,06-B,07-D,08-A,09-B,10-B,11-D,12-C,13-B,14-D,
15-B,16-A,17-D,18-B,19-D,20-A,21-C

25. Drugs for Angina Pectoris treatment

1. Angina pectoris is:
a) Severe constricting chest pain, often radiating from the precordium to the left shoulder and down the arm,due to insufficient blood supply to the heart that is usually caused by coronary disease
b) An often fatal form of arrhythmia characterized by rapid, irregular fibrillar twitching of the ventricles of the heart instead
of normal contractions, resulting in a loss of pulse
c) The cardiovascular condition in which the heart ability to pump blood weakens
d) All of the above

2. All these drug groups useful in angina both decrease myocardial oxygen requirement (by decreasing the determinationsof oxygen demand) and increase myocardial oxygen delivery (by reversing coronary arterial spasm), EXCEPT:
a) Nitrates and nitrite drugs (Nitroglycerin, Isosorbide dinitrate)
b) Calcium channel blockers (Nifedipine, Nimodipine)
c) Beta-adrenoceptor-blocking drugs (Atenolol, Metoprolol)
d) Potassium channel openers (Minoxidil)

3. This drug group useful in angina decreases myocardial oxygen requirement (by decreasing the determinations of oxygendemand) and does not increase maycardial oxygen delivery (by reversing coronary arterial spasm):
a) Nitrates and nitrite drugs (Nitroglycerin, Isosorbide dinitrate)
b) Myotropic coronary dilators (Dipyridamole)
c) Potassium channel openers (Minoxidil)
d) Beta-adrenoceptor-blocking drugs (Atenolol, Mtoprolol)

4. This drug group useful in angina increase myocardial oxygen delivery (by-reversing coronary arterial spasm) and does not decrease myocardial oxygen requirement (by decreasing the determinations of oxygen demand):
a) Beta-adrenoceptor-blocking drugs (Atenolol, Metoprolol):
b) Myotropic coronary dilators (Dipyridamole)
c) Calcium channel blockers (Nifedipine, Nimodipine)
d) Potassium channel openers (Minoxidil)

5. Which of the following statements concerning nitrate mechanism of action is True?

a) Therapeutically active agents in this group are capable of releasing nitric oxide (NO) in to vascular smooth muscle target tissues

b) Nitric oxide (NO) is an effective activator of soluble guanylyl cyclase and probably acts mainly through this mechanism

c) Nitrates useful in angina decrease myocardial oxygen requirement (by decreasing the determinations of oxygen demand) and increase myocardial oxygen delivery (by reversing coronary arterial spasm)

d) All of the above

6. Which of the following nitrates and nitrite drugs are long-acting?

a) Nitroglycerin, sublingual

b) Isosorbide dinitrate, sublingual (Isordil, Sorbitrate)

c) Amyl nitrite, inhalant (Aspirols, Vaporole)

d) Sustac

7. Which of the following nitrates and nitrite drugs is a short-acting drug?

a) Nitroglycerin, 2% ointment (Nitrol)

b) Nitroglycerin, oral sustained-release (Nitrong)

c) Amyl nitrite, inhalant (Aspirols, Vaporole)

d) Sustac

8. Which of the following nitrates and nitrite drugs is used for prevention of angina attack?

a) Nitroglycerin, 2% ointment (Nitrol)

b) Nitroglycerin, oral sustained-release (Nitrong)

c) Isosorbide mononitrate (Ismo)

d) All of the above

9. Duration of nitroglycerin action (sublingual) is:

a) 10-30 minutes

b) 6-8 hours

c) 3-5 minutes

d) 1.5-2 hours

10. The following statements concerning mechanism of nitrate beneficial clinical effect are true, EXCEPT?

a) Decreased myocardial oxygen requirement

b) Relief of coronary artery spasm

c) Improved perfusion to ischemic myocardium

d) Increased myocardial oxygen consumption

11. Side effect of nitrates and nitrite drugs are, EXCEPT:
a) Orthostatic hypotension, tachycardia
b) GI disturbance
c) Throbbing headache
d) Tolerance

12. The following statements concerning mechanism of calcium channel blockers' action are true, EXCEPT:
a) Therapeutically active agents in this group are capable of releasing nitric oxide (NO) in vascular smooth muscle target tissues
b) Calcium channel blockers bind to L-type calcium channel sites
c) Calcium channel blockers useful in angina decrease myocardial oxygen requirement (by decreasing the determinations of oxygen demand) and increase myocardial oxygen delivery (by reversing coronary arterial spasm)
d) Calcium channel blockers decrease transmembrane calcium current associated in smooth muscle with long-lasting relaxation and in a cardiac muscle with a reduction in contractility

13. Which of the following antianginal agents is a calcium channel blocker?
a) Nitroglycerin
b) Dipyridamole
c) Minoxidil
d) Nifedipine

14. Which of the following cardiovascular system effects refers to a calcium channel blocker?
a) The reduction of peripheral vascular resistance
b) The reduction of cardiac contractility and, in some cases, cardiac output
c) Relief of coronary artery spasm
d) All of the above

15. Main clinical use of calcium channel blockers is:
a) Angina pectoris
b) Hypertension
c) Supraventricular tachyarrhythmias
d) All of the above

16. Which of the following antianginal agents is a myotropic coronary dilator:
a) Dipyridamole
b) Validol
c) Atenolol
d) Alinidine

17. Which of the following antianginal agents is a beta-adrenoceptor-blocking drug:
a) Dipyridamole
b) Validol
c) Atenolol
d) Alinidine

18. The following agents are cardioselective beta1-adrenoceptor-blocking drugs labeled for use in angina, EXCEPT:
a) Metoprolol
b) Talinolol
c) Atenolol
d) Propranolol

19. Which of the following statements concerning beta-adrenoceptor-blocking drugs are true:
a) These agents decrease transmembrane calcium current associated in a smooth muscle with long-lasting relaxation and in a cardiac muscle with a reduction in contractility
b) These agents has a moderate reflex and vascular dilative action caused by the stimulation of sensitive nerve endings
c) Beneficial effects of these agents are related primarily to their hemodynamic effects – decreased heart rate,blood pressure, and contractility – which decrease myocardial oxygen requirements at rest and during exercise
d) These agents increase the permeability of K channels, probably ATP - dependent K channels, that results in stabilizing the membrane potential of excitable cells near the resting potential

20. Which of the following antianginal agents refers to reflex coronary dilators:
a) Dipyridamole
b) Validol
c) Atenolol
d) Alinidine

21. Which of the following statements concerning Validol is true:
a) Validol has a moderate reflex and vascular dilative action caused by the stimulation of sensitive nerve endings
b) At sublingual administration the effect is produced in five minutes and 70 % of the preparation is released in 3 minutes

c) It is used in cases of angina pectoris, motion sickness, nausea, vomiting when seasick or airsick and headaches due to taking nitrates
d) All of the above

22. Which of the following antianginal agents is the specific bradycardic drug:
a) Dipyridamole
b) Validol
c) Atenolol
d) Alinidine

23. Following statements concerning specific bradycardic agents (Falipamil, Alinidine) are true, EXCEPT:
a) Bradycardic drugs have a moderate reflex and vascular dilative action caused by the stimulation of sensitivenerve endings
b) The predominant effect of bradycardic drugs is a decrease in heart rate without significant changes in arterial pressure
c) The protective effect of bradycardic drugs is likely due to a reduced O_2demand
d) Specific bradycardic agents are used in the management of a wide range of cardiovascular disorders, including sinus tachyarrhythmias and angina pectoris

24. Which of the following statements concerning Dipyridamole is true?
a) Dipyridamole is an agent that blocks the reabsorption and breakdown of adenosine that results in an increase of endogenous adenosine and vasodilatation
b) The drug causes relative hypoperfusion of myocardial regions served by coronary arteries with haemodynamically significant stenoses
c) Dipyridamole is a platelet aggregation inhibitor
d) All of the above

25. Which of the following antianginal agents is a potassium channel opener:
a) Dipyridamole
b) Validol
c) Atenolol
d) Minoxidil

26. Which of the following statements concerning potassium channel openers is true?

a) These agents decrease transmembrane calcium current associated in a smooth muscle with long-lasting relaxationand in a cardiac muscle with a reduction in contractility

b) These agents has a moderate reflex and vascular dilative action caused by the stimulation of sensitive nerve endings

c) Beneficial effects of these agents are related primarily to their hemodynamic effects – decreased heart rate, blood pressure, and contractility – which decrease myocardial oxygen requirements at rest and during exercise

d) These agents increase the permeability of K channels, probably ATP- ATP- dependent K channels, that results in stabilizing the membrane potential of excitable cells near the resting potential

Answer Key

01-A,02-C,03-D,04-B,06-D,07-C,08-D,09-A,10-D,11-B,12-A,13-D,14-D,15-D, 16-A,17-C,18-D,19-C,20-B,21-D,22-D,23-A,24-D,25-D,26-D

26. Antihypertensive drugs

1. This drug reduces blood pressure by acting on vasomotor centers in the CNS:
a) Labetalol
b) Clonidine
c) Enalapril
d) Nifedipine

2. All of the following are central acting antihypertensive drugs EXCEPT:
a) Methyldopa
b) Clonidine
c) Moxonidine
d) Minoxidil

3. A ganglioblocking drug for hypertension treatment is:
a) Hydralazine
b) Tubocurarine
c) Trimethaphan
d) Metoprolol

4. Pick out the sympatholythic drug:
a) Labetalol
b) Prazosin
c) Guanethidine
d) Clonidine

5. Tick the drug with nonselective beta-adrenoblocking activity:
a) Atenolol
b) Propranolol
c) Metoprolol
d) Nebivolol

6. Choose the selective blocker of beta-1 adrenoreceptors:
a) Labetalol
b) Prazosin
c) Atenolol
d) Propranolol

7. Pick out the drug – an alpha and beta adrenoreceptors blocker:
a) Labetalol
b) Verapamil
c) Nifedipine
d) Metoprolol

8. This drug inhibits the angiotensin-converting enzyme:
a) Captopril
b) Enalapril
c) Ramipril
d) All of the above

9. This drug is a directly acting vasodilator:
a) Labetalol
b) Clonidine
c) Enalapril
d) Nifedipine

10. Pick out the diuretic agent for hypertension treatment:
a) Losartan
b) Dichlothiazide
c) Captopril
d) Prazosin

11. This drug blocks alpha-1 adrenergic receptors:
a) Prazosin
b) Clonidine
c) Enalapril
d) Nifedipine

12. This drug activates alpha-2 adrenergic receptors:
a) Labetalol
b) Phentolamine
c) Clonidine
d) Enalapril

13. This drug is an inhibitor of renin synthesis:
a) Propranolol
b) Enalapril
c) Diazoxide
d) Losartan

14. This drug is a non-peptide angiotensin II receptor antagonist:
a) Clonidine
b) Captopril
c) Losartan
d) Diazoxide

15. This drug is a potassium channel activator:
a) Nifedipine
b) Saralasin
c) Diazoxide
d) Losartan

16. All of the following statements regarding angiotensin II are true EXCEPT:
a) It is a peptide hormone
b) It stimulates the secretion of aldosterone
c) Angiotensin I is almost as potent as angiotensin II
d) It is a potent vasoconstrictor

17. This drug is contraindicated in patients with bronchial asthma:
a) Propranolol
b) Clonidine
c) Enalapril
d) Nifedipine

18. This drug is converted to an active metabolite after absorption:
a) Labetalol
b) Clonidine
c) Enalapril
d) Nifedipine

19. This drug routinely produces some tachycardia:
a) Propranolol
b) Clonidine
c) Enalapril
d) Nifedipine

20. All of the following statements regarding vasodilators are true EXCEPT:
a) Hydralazine causes tachycardia
b) Nifedipine is a dopamine receptor antagonist
c) Nitroprusside dilates both arterioles and veins
d) Minoxidil can cause hypertrichosis

21. All of the following statements regarding verapamil are true EXCEPT:
a) It blocks L-type calcium channels
b) It increases heart rate
c) It relaxes coronary artery smooth muscle
d) It depresses cardiac contractility

22. Choose the unwanted effects of clonidine:
a) Parkinson's syndrome
b) Sedative and hypnotic effects
c) Agranulocytosis and aplastic anemia
d) Dry cough and respiratory depression

23. The reason of beta-blockers administration for hypertension treatment is:
a) Peripheral vasodilatation
b) Diminishing of blood volume
c) Decreasing of heart work
d) Depression of vasomotor center

24. An endogenous vasoconstrictor that can stimulate aldosterone release from suprarenal glands:
a) Angiotensinogen
b) Angiotensin I
c) Angiotensin II
d) Angiotensin-converting enzyme

25. Choose the group of antihypertensive drugs which diminishes the metabolism of bradykinin:
a) Ganglioblockers
b) Alfa-adrenoblockers
c) Angiotensin-converting enzyme inhibitors
d) Diuretics

26. Hydralazine (a vasodilator) can produce:
a) Seizures, extrapyramidal disturbances
b) Tachycardia, lupus erhythromatosis
c) Acute hepatitis
d) Aplastic anemia

27. Choose the vasodilator which releases NO:
a) Nifedipine
b) Hydralazine
c) Minoxidil
d) Sodium nitroprusside

28. The reason of diuretics administration for hypertension treatment is:
a) Block the adrenergic transmission
b) Diminishing of blood volume and amount of Na+ ions in the vessels
   endothelium
c) Depression of rennin-angiotensin-aldosterone system
d) Depression of the vasomotor center

29. Tick the diuretic agent – aldosterone antagonist:
a) Furosemide
b) Spironolactone
c) Dichlothiazide
d) Captopril

30. Tick the diuretic agent having a potent and rapid effect:
a) Furosemide
b) Spironolactone
c) Dichlothiazide
d) Indapamide

Answer Key

01-B,02-D,03-C,04-C,05-B,06-C,07-A,08-D,09-D,10-B,11-A,12-C,13-A,14-C,
15-C,16-C,17-A,18-C,19-D,20-B,21-B,22-B,23-C,24-C,25-C-26-B,27-D,28-B,29-B,30-A

27. Hypertensive (anti-hypotensive) drugs. Drugs influencing cerebral blood flow. Anti-migraine agents

1. The main principle of shock treatment is:
a) To increase the arterial pressure
b) To increase the peripheral vascular resistance
c) To increase the cardiac output
d) To improve the peripheral blood flow

2. Pick out the drug which increases cardiac output:
a) Noradrenalin
b) Methyldopa
c) Phenylephrine
d) Angiotensinamide

3. Tick the synthetic vasoconstrictor having an adrenomimic effect:
a) Noradrenalin
b) Adrenalin
c) Phenylephrine
d) Angiotensinamide

4. Indicate the vasoconstrictor of endogenous origin:
a) Ephedrine
b) Phenylephrine
c) Xylomethazoline
d) Angiotensinamide

5. Which type of receptors can be activated by angiotensinamide:
a) Adrenergic receptors
b) Cholinergic receptors
c) Dopaminergic receptors
d) Angiotensin's receptors

6. General unwanted effects of vasoconstrictors is:
a) Increase of arterial pressure
b) Increase of cardiac output
c) Decrease of peripheral blood flow
d) Increase of blood volume

7. For increasing blood pressure in case of low cardiac output the following agents must be used:
a) Ganglioblockers
b) Vasoconstrictors
c) Positive inotropic drugs
d) Diuretics

8. Tick the positive inotropic drug of glycoside structure:
a) Dopamine
b) Digoxin
c) Dobutamine
d) Adrenalin

9. Tick the positive inotropic drug of non-glycoside structure:
a) Digitoxin
b) Digoxin
c) Dobutamine
d) Strophanthin

10. Dopamine at low doses influences mainly:
a) Alfa-adrenoreceptors (leads to peripheral vasoconstriction)
b) Dopamine receptors (leads to vasodilation of renal and mesenterial vessels)
c) Beta-1 adrenoreceptors (leads to enhanced cardiac output)
d) All of the above

11. Dopamine at medium doses influences mainly:
a) Alfa-adrenoreceptors (leads to peripheral vasoconstriction)
b) Dopamine receptors (leads to vasodilation of renal and mesenterial vessels)
c) Beta-1 adrenoreceptors (leads to enhanced cardiac output)
d) All of the above

12. Dopamine in high doses influences mainly the:
a) Alfa-adrenoreceptors (leads to peripheral vasoconstriction)
b) Dopamine's receptors (leads to vasodilation of renal and mesenterial vessels)
c) Beta-1 adrenoreceptors (leads to enhancing of cardiac output)
d) All of the above

13. Tick the group of drugs for treatment of shock with hypovolaemia (reduced circulating blood volume):
a) Positive inotropic drugs
b) Vasoconstrictors
c) Plasmoexpanders
d) Analeptics and tonics

14. Tick the group of drugs for chronic hypotension treatment:
a) Positive inotropic drugs
b) Vasoconstrictors
c) Plasmoexpanders
d) Analeptics and tonics

15. Indicate the group of drugs influencing the cerebral flow:
a) Ca-channel blockers
b) Derivatives of GABA
c) Derivatives of Vinca minor plant
d) All the above

16. Tick the drug influencing the blood flow which is related to antiplatelet agents:
a) Heparin
b) Aspirin
c) Pyracetam
d) Tanakan

17. Which of the following drugs is related to anticoagulants and may be useful in disorders of cerebral circulation?
a) Aspirin
b) Cinnarizine
c) Nicergoline
d) Heparin

18. Indicate the drugs which are Ca-channel blockers influencing the brain blood flow:
a) Aminalon, Picamilon
b) Nimodipine, Cinnarizine
c) Heparin, Warfarin
d) Vinpocetine, Nicergoline

19. Indicate the drugs influencing the blood flow in the brain - derivatives of GABA:
a) Aminalon, Picamilon
b) Nimodipine, Cinnarizine
c) Heparin, Warfarin
d) Vinpocetine, Nicergoline

20. Indicate the drug - Vinca minor alcaloid:
a) Nicergoline
b) Warfarin
c) Cinnarizine
d) Vinpocetine

21. Tick the drug – a derivative of Ergot:
a) Nicergoline
b) Warfarin
c) Cinnarizine
d) Vinpocetine

22. Indicate the nootropic agent useful in disorders of brain circulation:
a) Aspirin
b) Pyracetam
c) Warfarin
d) All the above

23. What is the main action of GABA derivatives in disorders of brain circulation?
a) Decrease of vessel permeability
b) Stimulation of the metabolic processes in neurons
c) Brain vessel constriction
d) Intracranial pressure increase

24. Choose the appropriate mechanism of vinpocetine action:
a) It dilates cerebral vessels and improves blood supply
b) It constricts cerebral vessels and decreases blood supply
c) It stimulates GABA-receptors and thus increases cerebral metabolic processes
d) It constricts peripheral vessels and increases blood pressure

25. Antiaggregants are used in disorders of brain circulation for:
a) Stimulation of the metabolic processes in neurons
b) Dilation of cerebral vessels
c) Improving the microcirculation in cerebral tissue
d) All the above

26. Migraine is a disorder connected with:
a) Thrombosis of cerebral vessels
b) Brain hemorrhage
c) Dysfunction of regulation of cerebral vessel tonus
d) Malignant growth in brain

27. The following Indol derivative is used for treatment of acute migraine attack:
a) Paracetamol
b) Sumatriptan
c) Ergotamine
d) Metoclopramide

28. The following Ergot derivative is used for treatment of acute migraine attack:
a) Paracetamol
b) Sumatriptan
c) Ergotamine
d) Metoclopramide

29. The derivative of lysergic acid for migraine attacke prevention is :
a) Metoclopramide
b) Methysergide
c) Sumatriptan
d) Ergotamine

Answer Key

01-D,02-A,03-C,04-D,05-D,06-C,07-C,08-B,09-C,10-B,11-C,12-A,13-C,14-D,15-D,16-B,17-D,18-B,19-A,20-D,21-A,22-B,23-B,24-A,25-C,26-C,27-B,28-C,29-B

28. Hypothalamic & Pituitary Hormones, Thyroid & Antithyroid Drugs

1. Hormones are:
a) Products of endocrine gland secretion
b) Mediators of inflammatory process
c) By-products of tissue metabolism
d) Product of exocrine gland secretion

2. Select an endocrine drug which is an amino acid derivative:
a) Insulin
b) Hydrocortisone
c) Calcitonin
d) Thyroxine

3. Select an endocrine drug which is a peptide derivative:
a) Oxitocin
b) Prednisolone
c) Nandrolone
d) Progesterone

4. Select an endocrine drug which is a steroidal derivative:
a) Gonadorelin
b) Insulin
c) Levothyroxine
d) Hydrocortisone

5. Hormone analogues are:
a) Naturally occurring substances but slightly different from hormones
b) Naturally occurring substances but less efficacious than hormones
c) Naturally occurring substances having the same structure but different Pharmacological properties than hormones
d) Synthetic compounds, which resemble the naturally occurring hormones

6. Regarding the mechanism of action of hormones, indicate the FALSE statement:
a) Hormones interact with the specific receptors in the wall of the cells

b) Cyclic AMP acts as a second messenger system

c) They stimulate adenylcyclase enzyme

d) Many hormones owe their effect to primary actions on subcellular membrane.

7. Hypothalamic and pituitary hormones (and their synthetic analogs) have pharmacologic applications in three areas,EXCEPT the following:

a) As replacement therapy for hormone deficiency states

b) As drug therapy for a variety of disorders using pharmacologic doses to elicit a hormonal effect that is not present at physiologic a blood levels

c) As a diagnostic tool for performing stimulation tests to diagnose hypo- or hyperfunctional endocrine states

d) As food supplements

8. Which of the following hormones is produced by the hypothalamic gland?

a) Growth hormone-releasing hormone (GHRH)

b) Follicle-stimulating hormone (FSH)

c) Aldosterone

d) Estradiol

9. Which of the following hormones is produced by the anterior lobe of the pituitary?

a) Thyrotropin-releasing hormone (TRH)

b) Corticotropin-releasing hormone (CRH)

c) Growth hormone (somatotropin, GH)

d) Growth hormone-releasing hormone (GHRH)

10. The posterior pitutary does NOT secret:

a) Vasopressin

b) Oxytocin

c) Growth hormone

d) All of the above

11. Which of the following organs is a target for prolactin?

a) Liver

b) Adrenal cortex

c) Thyroid

d) Mammary gland

12. Which of the following organ hormones is a target for growth hormone (somatotropine, GH)?

a) Glucocorticoids

b) Insulin-like growth factors (IGF, somatomedins)

c) Triiodthyronine
d) Testosterone

13. All of the following statements about growth hormone are true, EXCEPT:
a) It may stimulate the synthesis or release of somatomedins
b) Low levels of insulin-like growth factor (IGF)-1 are associated with dwarfism
c) Hypersecretion can result in acromegaly
d) It is contraindicated in subjects with closed epiphyses

14. Correct statments about adrenocorticotropic hormone (ACTH) include all of the following ,except:
a) Endogenous ACTH is also called corticotropin
b) ACTH stimulates the synthesis of corticosteroids
c) ACTH is most useful clinically as a diagnostic tool in adrenal insufficiency
d) The oral route is the preferred rout of administration

15. Indications of bromocriptine are following, EXCEPT:
a) Prolactin-secreting adenomas
b) Amenorrhea-Galactorrhea
c) Prolactin deficiency
d) Acromegaly

16. Currently used dopamine agonists decreasing pituitary prolactin secretion are following:
a) Bromocriptine
b) Cabergoline
c) Pergolide
d) All of the above

17. Indications of oxitocin are following:
a) Labor and augment dysfunctional labor for conditions requiring early vaginal delivery
b) Incompleted abortion
c) For control of pospartum uterine hemorrhage
d) All of the above

18. Indications of vasopressin are following:
a) Diabetes mellitus
b) Hypertension
c) Pituitary diabetes insipidus
d) Incompleted abortion

19. Vasopressin possesses the following:
a) Antidiuretic property
b) Vasodilatation property
c) Release of a thyroid hormone into the plasma
d) Diuretic property

20. Oxytocin produces the following effects:
a) It causes contraction of the uterus
b) It assists the progress of spermatozoa into the uterine cavity
c) It brings about milk ejection from the lactating mammary gland
d) All of the above

21. Vasopressin causes a pressor effect by:
a) Releasing noradrenaline from the nerve terminals
b) Releasing and activating renin-angiotensin system
c) A direct action on smooth muscles of the blood vessels
d) All of the above mechanisms

22. Which of the following hormones is produced by the thyroid gland?
a) Thyroxine
b) Thyroid-stimulating hormone
c) Thyrotropin-releasing hormone
d) Thyroglobulin.

23. Which of the following hormones is produced by the thyroid gland?
a) Thyroid-stimulating hormone
b) Thyrotropin-releasing hormone
c) Triiodothyronine
d) Thyroglobulin.

24. Thyroid stimulating hormone regulates the following:
a) Iodine uptake
b) Biosynthesis of iodothyroglobulin
c) Release of thyroid hormone into the plasma
d) All of the above.

25. Thyroid hormones produce various pharmacological effects. Indicate the wrong statement(s).
a) Decline of the basal metabolic rate in the body
b) Increase in the rate and force of contraction of the heart
c) Increase in the blood cholestrol level
d) Increase in the heat production

26. Synthesis and release of thyroid hormones are controlled by:
a) Anterior pituitary alone
b) Hypothalamus alone
c) Blood levels of thyroid hormones alone
d) All of the above

27. Thyrotrophin stimulates the following processes:
a) Concentration of iodine by thyroid follicles
b) Iodination of thyroglobulin
c) Release of thyroxine and triidothyronine
d) De-iodination of thyroid hormones.

28. The rate of secretion of thyrotropin is controlled by:
a) The amount of iodine in the thyroid gland
b) The amount of thyroid hormones in the thyroid gland
c) The concentration of thyroid hormones in blood
d) The concentration of catecholamines in blood

29. Indications of thyroid hormones are following, EXCEPT:
a) Cretinism
b) Myxoedema
c) Hashimoto's disease
d) For treatment of simple obesity

30. The common side effect of thyroid hormones is following:
a) Increases in basal metabolic rate
b) Angina pectoris
c) Tremors
d) Exopthalmos

31. Currently used antithyroid drugs include the following, EXCEPT:
a) Propylthiouracil (PTU)
b) Diatrizoate sodium (Hypaque)
c) Methimazole (Tapazole)
d) Potassium perchlorate

32. In an area where goitre is endemic, which of the following drugs is used?
a) Iodide 1 part in 100000
b) Propylthiouracil 200 mg daily
c) Methimazole 40 mg daily
d) Any of the above can be used.

33. Iodide preparations can be used in following situations, EXCEPT:
a) In thyroid disorders
b) In granulomatous lesions e.g. Syphilis
c) As an antiseptic
d) In iodism

34. Daily administration of large doses (several milligrammes) of iodides to a thyrotoxic patient causes:
a) Involution of the thyroid which reaches a maximum in two weeks
b) Increased vascularity of the thyroid gland
c) Decreased storage of the colloid in the thyroid gland
d) Thyroid gland growing firm and less vascular

35. Radioiodines (I131 and I132) is suitable for:
a) Elderly patients (over 45 years)
b) Pregnant women
c) Nursing mothers
d) Younger patients

36. Radioiodines in the body emit:
a) Mainly β radiations
b) Mainly γ radiations
c) β and γ radiations equally.
d) Do not emit any radiation, therefore, are safe

Answer Key

01-A,02-D,03-A,04-D,05-D,06-A,07-D,08-A,09-C,10-C,11-D,12-B,13-C,14-D,
15-C,16-D,17-D,18-C,19-A,20-D,21-C,22-A,23-C,24-D,25-A,26-D,27-C,28-C,29-D,
30-D,31-D,32-A,33-D,34-D,35-A,36-A

29. Pancreatic Hormones & Antidiabetic Drugs

1. Secretory products of pancreatic β-cells are:
a) Glucagon, proglucagon
b) Insulin, C-peptide, proinsulin, islet amyloid polypeptide (IAPP)
c) Somatostatin
d) Pancreatic polypeptide (PP)

2. Insulin is:
a) A glycoprotein with a molecular weight of 6000
b) A small protein with a molecular weight of 5808 having disulphide linkage
c) A fructoolygosaccharide
d) A catecholamine

3. Insulin is a polypeptide hence:
a) It is resistant to destruction by gastric juice
b) It is destroyed by gastric juice
c) It is not a polypeptide
d) It is metabolized immediately by cellular enzymes

4. Insulin causes reduction in blood sugar level by the following mechanisms, EXCEPT:
a) Increased glucose uptake in the peripheral tissue
b) Reduction of breakdown of glycogen
c) Diminished gluconeogenesis
d) Decreased glucose absorption from the gut

5. Which of the following is true for glucagon?
a) Stimulates gluconeogenesis in the liver
b) Stimulates the secretion of insulin by beta cells
c) Inhibits glucose utilization by skeletal muscle
d) Inhibits uptake of aminoacids by cells.

6. Insulin can not be administered by:
a) Oral route
b) Intravenous route

c) Subcutaneous route

d) Intramuscular route.

7. Sources of human insulin production are:

a) Recombinant DNA techniques by inserting the proinsulin gene into *E. coli* or yeast

b) Postmortem insulin extraction from human autopsy pancreas

c) All of the above

d) None of the above

8. The primary reason for a physician to prescribe human insulin is that:

a) It has a faster onset of action than other insulins

b) It has a shorter duration of action than other insulins

c) It can be given to patients who have an allergy to animal insulins

d) It is more effective in preventing the complications of diabetes than animal insulins

9. Correct statements about crystalline zinc (regular) insulin include all of the following, EXCEPT:

a) It can serve as replacement therapy for juvenile-onset diabetes

b) It can be administered intravenously

c) It is a short-acting insulin

d) It can be administered orally

10. Diabetic coma is treated by the administration of:

a) Lente insulin

b) Glucose

c) Crystalline insulin

d) Oral anti-diabetic drugs.

11. Sulphonylureas act by:

a) Reducing the absorption of carbohydrate from the gut

b) Increasing the uptake of glucose in peripheral tissues

c) Reducing the hepatic gluconeogenesis

d) Stimulating the beta islet cells of pancreas to produce insulin

12. Currently used second-generation sulfonylureas include the following, EXCEPT:

a) Glyburide (Glibenclamide)

b) Glipizide (Glydiazinamide)

c) Glimepiride (Amaril)

d) Tolbutamide (Orinase)

13. Currently used oral hypoglycemic thiazolidinediones include the following, EXCEPT
a) Pioglitazone (Actos)
b) Rosiglitazone (Avandia)
c) Troglitazone (Rezulin)
d) All of the above

14. Thiazolidinediones act by:
a) Diminishing insulin resistance by increasing glucose uptake and metabolism in muscle and adipose tissues
b) Reducing the absorption of carbohydrate from the gut
c) Stimulating the beta islet cells of pancreas to produce insulin
d) All of the above

15. Currently used alpha-glucosidase inhibitors include the following, EXCEPT:
a) Pioglitazone (Actos)
b) Acarbose (Precose)
c) Miglitol (Glyset)
d) All of the above

16. Alpha-glucosidase inhibitors act by:
a) Diminishing insulin resistance by increasing glucose uptake and metabolism in muscle and adipose tissues
b) Competitive inhibiting of intestinal alpha ghucosidases and modulating the postprandial digestion and absorption of starch and disaccharides
c) Reducing the absorption of carbohydrate from the gut
d) Stimulating the beta islet cells of pancreas to produce insulin

17. Potency of action of
a) Miglitol is six times higher than that of acarbose
b) Acarbose is more than that of miglitol
c) Miglitol and acarbose is equal
d) Oral hypoglycemic agents depend on the severity of hyperglycemia

18. Which of the following oral hypoglycaemic drugs stimulates both synthesis and release of insulin from beta islet cells:
a) Glibenclamide
b) Phenformin
c) Buformine
d) Metformin

19. Currently used oral hypoglycemic biguanides include the following, EXCEPT:
a) Repaglinide (Prandin)
b) Metformin
c) Phenformine
d) Glipizide

20. The action of insulin is potentiated by:
a) Sulphonylureas
b) Glucagon
c) Biguanides
d) None of the above

21. Duration of action of:
a) Tolbutamide is more than that of chlorpropamide
b) Chlorpropamide is more than that of tolbutamide
c) Tolbutamide and chlorpropamide is equal
d) Oral hypoglycemic agents depend on the severity of hyperglycemia

22. Biguanides are used in the following conditions, EXCEPT:
a) As a supplement to sulphonylurea, where it is insufficient to give good results
b) In over weight diabetics
c) To reduce insulin requirements
d) In case of hyperglycemic shock

23. Which of the following agents is/are important hormonal antagonists of insulin in the body?
a) Glucagon
b) Adrenal steroids
c) Adrenaline
d) All of the above

24. Glucagon is:
a) A glycoprotein with a molecular weight of 6000
b) A peptide – identical in all mammals – consisting of a single chain of 29 amino acids
c) A a fructoolygosaccharide
d) A small protein with a molecular weight of 5808 having disulphide linkage

25. Which of the following statements is FALSE?
a) Glucagon is synthesized in the A cells of the pancreatic islets of Langerhans.

b) Glucagon is a peptide – identical in all mammals – consisting of a single chain of 29 amino acids

c) Glucagon is extensively degraded in the liver and kidney as well as in plasma, and at its tissue receptor sites.

d) Half-life of glucagon is between 6 and 8 hours, which is similar to that of insulin

26. Glucagon can be used in the following situations, EXCEPT:
a) Severe hypoglycemia
b) Severe hyperglycemia
c) Endocrine diagnosis
d) Beta-blocker poisoning

27. Main complications of insulin therapy include the following:
a) Hypoglycemia
b) Insulin allergy
c) Lipodystrophy at an injection site
d) All of the above

Answer Key
01-B,02-B,03-B,04-D,06-A,07-A,08-C,09-D,10-C,11-D,12-D,13-C,14-A,15-A,16-B,17-A,18-A,19-D,20-C,21-B,22-D,23-D,24-B,25-D,26-B,27-D

30. The Gonadal Hormones & Inhibitors

1. The major natural estrogens produced by women are following, EXCEPT:
a) Estradiol (Estradiol-17β, E_2)
b) Estron (E_1)
c) Ethinyl estradiol
d) Estriol (E_3)

2. Which of the following statements about estrogens are True:
a) Estrogens are required for normal sexual maturation and growth of the female
b) Estrogens decrease the rate of resorption of bone
c) Estrogens enhance the coagulability of blood
d) All of the above

3. The major synthetic estrogens are following, EXCEPT:
a) Dienestrol
b) Diethylstilbestrol
c) Benzestrol
d) Estradiol

4. Which of the following statements about estrogens are True:
a) Estradiol binds strongly to an α2-globulin and albumin with lower affinity
b) Estradiol is converted by liver and other tissues to estron and estriol and their 2-hydroxylated derivatives and conjugated metabolites and excreted in the bile
c) Estrone and estriol have lower affinity for the estrogen receptors than estradiol
d) All of the above

5. Indications of synthetic estrogens are following, EXCEPT:
a) Primary hypogonadism
b) Postmenopausal hormonal therapy
c) Hormonal contraception
d) For treatment of simple obesity

6. Main complications of estrogens' therapy include the following:
a) Postmenopausal uterine bleeding
b) Breast tenderness
c) Hyperpigmentation
d) All of the above

7. Main contraindications of estrogens' therapy include the following:
a) Estrogen-dependent neoplasmas such as carcinoma of the endometrium or carcinoma of the breast
b) Undiagnosed genital bleeding
c) Liver disease
d) All of the above

8. Tamoxifen is:
a) Antiprogestin
b) Antiandrogen
c) Antiestrogen
d) Androgen

9. Progesterone is secreted by:
a) Ovarian follicles
b) Corpus luteum
c) Granulosa and theca cells
d) All of the above

10. The major natural progestin is:
a) Estradiol
b) Estron
c) Progesterone
d) Estriol

11. Which of the following statements about progestins is True:
a) Progesterone is rapidly absorbed following administration by any route
b) In the liver, progesterone is metabolized to pregnanediol and conjugated with glucuronic acid.
c) Significant amounts of progestins and their metabolites are excreted in the urine
d) All of the above

12. Noncontraceptive clinical uses of progestins are following:
a) Hormone replacement therapy
b) Dysmenorrhea
c) Endometriosis
d) All of the above

13. Mifepristone (RU-486) is:

a) Antiprogestin

b) Antiandrogen

c) Antiestrogen

d) Androgen

14. Actions of mifepristone (RU-486) include:

a) Inhibition of ovulation during the follicular phase by blocking hypothalamic-pituitary progesterone receptors, which suppresses midcycle gonadotropin release

b) During the luteal phase, inhibition of progesterone action on the uterus, which induces prostaglandin release from the endometrium

c) Termination of pregnancy by facilitating luteolysis, menstruation, uterine motility, softening of the cervix, and detachment of the embryo.

d) All of the above

15. All of the following statements about oral contraceptives are true, EXCEPT:

a) The "combination pill" contains both estrogen and progestin

b) Ethinyl estradiol and mestranol are commonly used in oral contraceptives

c) The "minipill" contains progestin alone

d) The "triphasic pill" contains estrogen, progestin, and luteinizing hormine (LH)

Answer Key

01-C,02-D,03-D,04-D,05-D,06-D,07-D,08-C,09-B,10-C,11-D,12-D,13-A,14-D, 15-D

31. Glucocorticoid, Steroidal & Nonsteroidal Anti-Inflammatory Drugs

1. Glucocorticoids are hormonal steroids:
a) Having an important effect on intermediary metabolism, cardiovascular function, growth, and immunity
b) Having principally salt-retaining activity
c) Having androgenic or estrogenic activity
d) All of the above

2. Inflammation is:
a) A localized protective reaction of a tissue to irritation, injury, or infection, characterized by pain, redness,swelling, and sometimes loss of function
b) A deficiency of the normal immune response.
c) A reaction resulting from an immune reaction produced by an individual's white blood cells or antibodies acting on the body's own tissues or extracellular proteins.
d) All of the above

3. An acute, transient phase, of inflammation is characterized by:
a) Local vasodilatation and increased capillary permeability (phase of damage)
b) Infiltration of leucocytes and phagocytic cells (phase of exudation)
c) Tissue degeneration and fibrosis occurrence (phase of proliferation)
d) All of the above

4. A delayed, subacute phase, of inflammation is characterized by:
a) Local vasodilatation and increased capillary permeability (phase of damage)
b) Infiltration of leucocytes and phagocytic cells (phase of exudation)
c) Tissue degeneration and fibrosis occurrence (phase of proliferation)
d) All of the above

5. A chronic, proliferative phase, of inflammation is characterized by:
a) Local vasodilatation and increased capillary permeability (phase of damage)
b) Infiltration of leucocytes and phagocytic cells (phase of exudation)
c) Tissue degeneration and fibrosis occurrence (phase of proliferation)
d) All of the above

6. The following substances are considered to be referred to as eicosanoids:
a) Prostaglandins
b) Leukotrienes
c) Thromboxanes
d) All of the above

7. Correct statements about cortisol (hydrocortisone) include all of the following, EXCEPT:
a) Cortisol is synthesized from cholesterol
b) ACTH governs cortisol secretion
c) Most cortisol is inactivated in the liver
d) The half-life of cortisol in the circulations is normally about 60-90 hours.

8. Correct statements about glucocorticoids include all of the following, EXCEPT:
a) Effects of glucocorticoids are mediated by widely distributed glucocorticoid receptors that are members of the superfamily of nuclear receptors.
b) Glucocorticoids have dose-related metabolic effects on carbohydrate, protein, and fat metabolism.
c) Glucocorticoids have pro-inflammatory effects.
d) Glucocorticoids have catabolic effects in lymphoid and connective tissue, muscle, fat, and skin.

9. Physiologic doses of glucocorticoid can result in:
a) Increased liver glycogen stores, gluconeogenesis and lipolysis
b) Maintenance of cardiovascular function (by potentiation of norepinephrine) and skeletal muscle function
c) Increased hemoglobin synthesis, resulting in elevated of red blood cell count
d) All of the above

10. Which of the following glucocorticoids is a short- to medium-acting drug?
a) Prednisolon
b) Dexamethasone
c) Triamcinolone
d) All of the above

11. Which of the following glucocorticoids is an intermediate-acting drug?
a) Cortisone
b) Triamcinolone
c) Butamethasone
d) All of the above

12. Which of the following glucocorticoids is a long-acting drug?
a) Prednisolon
b) Dexamethasone
c) Triamcinolone
d) All of the above

13. Which of the following glucocorticoids have one fluoride atom in its chemical structure?
a) Prednisolon
b) Fluocinolone
c) Triamcinolone
d) All of the above

14. Which of the following glucocorticoids have two fluoride atoms in its chemical structure?
a) Prednisolon
b) Dexamethasone
c) Fluocinolone
d) Triamcinolone

15. Which of the following glucocorticoids has no fluoride atoms in its chemical structure?
a) Prednisolon
b) Dexamethasone
c) Fluocinolone
d) Triamcinolone

16. Anti-inflammatory effect of glucocorticoids is caused by
a) Reducing the prostaglandin and leukotriene which results from inhibition of phospholipase A
b) Reducing macrophages migration into the site of inflammation
c) Decreasing capillary permeability
d) All of the above

17. Which of the following statements concerning the anti-inflammatory effect of glucocorticoids is TRUE?
a) Anti-inflammatory effect of glucocorticoids results from inhibition of cyclooxygenase
b) Anti-inflammatory effect of glucocorticoids results from inhibition of phospholipase A_2 and reducing prostaglandin and leukotriene synthesis

c) Induction of cyclooxygenase II expression which results in reducing amount of an enzyme available to produce prostoglandins

d) All of the above

18. Immunosupressive effect of glucocorticoids is caused by:

a) Reducing concentration of lymphocytes (T and B cells) and inhibiting function of tissue macrophages and other antigen-presenting cells

b) Suppression of cyclooxygenase II expression which results in reducing amount of an enzyme available to produce prostoglandins

c) Activation of phospholipase A_2 and reducing prostaglandin and leukotriene synthesis.

d) All of the above

19. Which of the following statements concerning the anti-inflammatory effect of NSAIDs are TRUE?

a) Anti-inflammatory effect of NSAIDs results from inhibition of cyclooxygenase

b) Anti-inflammatory effect of NSAIDs results from inhibition of phospholipase A_2 and reducing prostaglandin and leukotriene synthesis

c) Anti-inflammatory effect of NSAIDs results from induction of cyclooxygenase II expression which results in reducing the amount of an enzyme available to produce prostoglandins

d) All of the above

20. Indication of glucocorticoids is:

a) Chronic (Addison's disease) and acute adrenocortical insufficiency

b) Organ transplants (prevention and treatment of rejection – immunosuppression)

c) Inflammatory conditions of bones and joints (arthritis, bursitis, tenosynovitis).

d) All of the above

21. Indications of glucocorticoids are following, EXCEPT:

a) Gastrointestinal diseases (inflammatory bowel disease)

b) Postmenopausal hormonal therapy

c) Inflammatory conditions of bones and joints (arthritis, bursitis, tenosynovitis)

d) Skin diseases (atopic dermatitis, dermatoses, localized neurodermatitis)

22. Serious side effects of glucocorticoids include the following, EXCEPT:

a) Acute peptic ulcers

b) Iatrogenic Cushing's syndrome (rounding, puffiness, fat deposition and plethora alter the appearance of the face –moon faces)

c) Salicylism (vomiting, tinnitus, decreased hearing, and vertigo)

d) Hypomania or acute psychosis

23. Serious side effects of glucocorticoids include the following:
a) Adrenal suppression
b) Insomnia, behavioral changes (primarily hypomania)
c) Rounding, puffiness, fat deposition and plethora alter the appearance of the face – moon faces
d) All of the above

24. Which of the following property combinations is peculiar to the majority of NSAIDs?
a) Antihistaminic, antipyretic, analgesic
b) Immunodepressive, anti-inflammatory, analgesic
c) Antipyretic, analgesic, anti-inflammatory
d) Anti-inflammatory, immunodepressive, antihistaminic

25. Which of the following NSAIDs is a propionic acid derivative?
a) Ibuprofen
b) Indomethacin
c) Metamizole (Analgin)
d) Diclofenac

26. Which of the following NSAIDs is an indol derivative?
a) Ibuprofen
b) Indomethacin
c) Meclofenamic acid
d) Diclofenac

27. Which of the following NSAIDs is a pyrazolone derivative?
a) Ibuprofen
b) Indomethacin
c) Metamizole (Analgin)
d) Diclofenac

28. Which of the following NSAIDs is a fenamate derivative?
a) Phenylbutazone
b) Indomethacin
c) Meclofenamic acid
d) Diclofenac

29. Which of the following NSAIDs is an oxicam derivative?
a) Piroxicam
b) Indomethacin
c) Meclofenamic acid
d) Diclofenac

30. Which of the following NSAIDs is a selective COX-2 inhibitor?
a) Piroxicam
b) Indomethacin
c) Celecoxib
d) Diclofenac

31. Which of the following NSAIDs is a nonselective COX inhibitor
a) Piroxicam
b) Rofecoxib
c) Celecoxib
d) All of the above

32. The following statements concerning aspirin are true, EXCEPT:
a) In contrast to most other NSAIDs, aspirin irreversibly inhibits COX
b) Aspirin interferes with the chemical mediators of the kallikrein system
c) Aspirin inhibits phospholipase A_2
d) Aspirin inhibits tromboxane A_2 formation

33. Indication for aspirin administration are the following, EXCEPT:
a) Inflammatory conditions
b) Decreasing the incidence of transient ischemic attack, unstable angina, coronary artery thrombosis with myocardial infarction, and thrombosis after coronary artery bypass grafting
c) Relieving severe visceral pain, e.g. myocardial infarction, cancer pain condition, renal or biliary colic
d) Reducing elevated body temperature

34. Side effects of aspirin include following:
a) Gastric upset (intolerance)
b) Salicylism (vomiting, tinnitus, decreased hearing, and vertigo)
c) Gastric ulcers and upper gastrointestinal bleeding
d) All of the above

35. Serious side effects of metamizole (analgin) include the following:
a) Agranulocytosis, aplastic anemia
b) Salicylism (vomiting, tinnitus, decreased hearing, and vertigo)
c) Iatrogenic Cushing's syndrome (rounding, puffiness, fat deposition and plethora alter the appearance of the face –moon faces)
d) All of the above

36. Side effects of indometacin include the following:
a) Abdominal pain, diarrhea, gastrointestinal hemorrhage and pancreatitis
b) Dizziness, confusion and depression
c) Trombocytopenia
d) All of the above

37. Which of the following drugs is a 5-lipoxygenase (5-LOG) inhibitor?
a) Ibuprofen
b) Zileuton (Zyflo)
c) Metamizole (Analgin)
d) Diclofenac

38. Which of the following drugs is a leucotreine D4 receptor (LTD4) blocker?
a) Ibuprofen
b) Zileuton (Zyflo)
c) Zafirleukast (Accolate)
d) Diclofenac

39. Which of the following drugs is a thromboxane A2 receptor (TXA2) antagonist?
a) Sulotroban
b) Zileuton (Zyflo)
c) Zafirleukast (Accolate)
d) Diclofenac

Answer Key

01-A,02-A,03-A,04-B,05-C,06-D,07-D,08-C,09-D,10-A,11-B,11-B,13-C,14-C,15-A,16-D,17-B,18-A,19-A,20-D,21-B,22-C,23-D,24-C,25-A,26-B,27-C,28-C,29-A,30-A,31-A,32-C,33-C,34-D,35-A,36-D,37-B,38-C,39-A

32. Immunotropic & Antiallergic Agents

1. Immunodeficiency:
a) A localized protective reaction of tissue to irritation, injury, or infection, characterized by pain, redness, swelling, and sometimes a loss of function
b) A disorder or deficiency of the normal immune response
c) A disease resulting from an immune reaction produced by an individual's white blood cells or antibodies acting on the body's own tissues or extracellular proteins
d) All of the above

2. H1 histamine receptor subtype is distributed in:
a) Smooth muscle, endothelium and brain
b) Gastric mucosa, cardiac muscle, mast cells and brain
c) Presynaptically in brain, mesenteric plexus and other neurons
d) All of the above

3. H2 histamine receptor subtype is distributed in:
a) Smooth muscle, endothelium and brain
b) Gastric mucosa, cardiac muscle, mast cells and brain
c) Presynaptically in brain, mesenteric plexus and other neurons
d) All of the above

4. Most tissue histamine is sequestered and bound in:
a) Granules in mast cells or basophils
b) Cell bodies of histaminergic neurons
c) Enterochromaffin-like cell of the fondus of the stomach
d) All of the above

5. These categories of histamine H1 antagonists are noted for sedative effects, EXCEPT:
a) Piperidines; i.e. Loratadine, Fexofenadine
b) Ethanolamines (aminoalkyl ethers); i.e. Dimedrol, Clistin
c) Ethylenediamines; i.e. Suprastine
d) Phenothiazines; i.e. Diprazine, Promethazine

6. Which category of histamine H1 antagonists is noted for the best antie-metic action?

a) Alkylamines (propylamines); i.e. Brompheniramine
b) Ethanolamines (aminoalkyl ethers); i.e. Doxylamine
c) Piperazines; i.e. Hydroxyzine, Cyclizine
d) Ethylenediamines; i.e. Suprastine

7. These categories of histamine H_1 antagonists are noted for the anticholinergic effect, EXCEPT:

a) Alkylamines (propylamines); i.e. Brompheniramine
b) Piperazines; i.e. Hydroxyzine, Cyclizine
c) Ethylenediamines; i.e. Suprastine
d) Phenothiazines; i.e. Diprazine, Promethazine

8. Which category of histamine H_1 antagonists is noted for the alpha-adrenoreceptor-blocking effect?

a) Alkylamines (propylamines); i.e. Brompheniramine
b) Ethanolamines (aminoalkyl ethers); i.e. Doxylamine, Dimedrol
c) Ethylenediamines; i.e. Suprastine
d) Phenothiazines; i.e. Diprazine, Promethazine

9. Which category of histamine H_1 antagonists is noted for the highest local anesthetic effect?

a) Alkylamines (propylamines); i.e. Brompheniramine
b) Piperidines; i.e. Loratadine, Fexofenadine
c) Ethylenediamines; i.e. Suprastine
d) Phenothiazines; i.e. Promethazine

10. Which category of histamine H_1 antagonists is recognized for as second-generation antihistamines?

a) Alkylamines (propylamines); i.e. Brompheniramine
b) Piperidines; i.e. Loratadine, Fexofenadine
c) Ethylenediamines; i.e. Suprastine
d) Phenothiazines; i.e. Promethazine

11. These histamine H_1 antagonists are recognized for as second-generation antihistamines, EXCEPT:

a) Astemizole
b) Loratadine (Claritin)
c) Cetirizine (Zyrtec)
d) Suprastine

12. Which of histamine H₁antagonists is noted for the serotonin-blocking effect?
a) Brompheniramine
b) Cyproheptadine
c) Suprastine
d) Dimedrol

13. Which of the following histamine H₁antagonists is a long-acting (up to 24-48 h) antihistamine drug?
a) Diazoline
b) Diprazine
c) Suprastine
d) Dimedrol

14. Which of histamine H₁antagonists is noted for the ulcerogenic effect?
a) Diazoline
b) Loratadine
c) Suprastine
d) Dimedrol

15. Indication for administration of histamine H₁antagonists is:
a) Prevention or treatment of the symptoms of allergic reactions
b) Motion sickness and vestibular disturbances
c) Nausea and vomiting in pregnancy ("morning sickness")
d) All of the above

16. Indications for administration of histamine H₁antagonists are the following EXCEPT:
a) Prevention or treatment of the symptoms of allergic reactions (rhinitis, urticaria)
b) Management of seizure states
c) Nausea and vomiting in pregnancy ("morning sickness")
d) Treatment of sleep disorders

17. Side effect of first-generation histamine H₁antagonists is:
a) Aplastic anemia
b) Vomiting, tinnitus, decreased hearing
c) Sedation
d) Gastric ulcers and upper gastrointestinal bleeding

18. Immunosupressive effect of glucocorticoids is caused by
a) Reducing concentration of lymphocytes (T and B cells) and inhibiting function of tissue macrophages and other antigen-presenting cells

b) Suppression of cyclooxygenase II expression that results in reducing amount of an enzyme available to produce prostoglandins

c) Activation of phospholipase A_2 and reducing prostaglandin and leukotriene synthesis

d) All of the above

19. Antiallergic effect of glucocorticoids is caused by:

a) Suppression of leukocyte migration and stabilizing lysosomal membranes

b) Reverse the capillary permeability associated with histamine release

c) Suppression of the immune response by inhibiting antibody synthesis

d) All of the above

20. The Immunosuppressive agent is:

a) Corticosteroids

b) Cyclosporine

c) Tacrolimus (FK 506)

d) All of the above

21. Class of cyclosporine A is:

a) Interferons

b) Immunosuppressive agents

c) Monoclonal antibodies

d) Immunoglobulins

22. Mechanism of action of cyclosporine A is:

a) Complement-mediated cytolysis of T lymphocytes

b) ADCC towards T lymphocytes

c) Inhibits calcineurin

d) Compete for Fc receptors with autoantibodies

23. Side effect of cyclosporine A is:

a) Tremor

b) GI disturbance

c) Hepatotoxicity

d) All of the above

24. Side effect of cyclosporine A is:

a) Tremor

b) Anorexia

c) Chills

d) Myalgia

25. Side effect of cyclosporine A is:
a) Diarrhea
b) Headache
c) GI disturbance
d) Immunosuppression

26. Indication of cyclosporine A is:
a) Secondary immunodeficiency
b) Hairy cell leukemia
c) Primary immunodeficiency
d) Idiopathic nephrotic syndrome

27. Half-life of cyclosporine A is:
a) 25-35 minutes
b) 21 days
c) 4 - 16 hours
d) 19 hours

28. Class of I.V. IgG preparation is:
a) Monoclonal antibodies
b) Immunosuppressive agents
c) Interferons
d) Immunoglobulins

29. Mechanism of action of I.V. IgG preparation is:
a) Inhibits CD3 receptor
b) Inhibits calcineurin
c) Complement-mediated cytolysis of T lymphocytes
d) Compete for Fc receptors with autoantibodies

30. Half-life of I.V. IgG preparation is:
a) 25-35 minutes
b) 19 hours
c) 4 - 16 hours
d) 21 days

31. Indication for I.V. IgG preparation administration is:
a) Kaposi's sarcoma
b) Acute rejection of organ transplant
c) Condyloma acuminatum
d) Prophylaxis of certain infections

32. Cytotoxic agents are the following EXCEPT:
a) Azathioprine
b) Cyclosporine
c) Leflunomide
d) Cyclophosphamide

33. Class of sirolimus (rapamycin) is:
a) Immunoglobulins
b) Interferons
c) Immunosuppressive agents
d) Monoclonal antibodies

34. Mechanism of action of sirolimus (rapamycin) is:
a) Anti-idiotype antibodies against autoantibodies
b) Modulation of CD3 receptor from the cell surface
c) Inhibits calcineurin
d) ADCC towards T lymphocytes

35. Monoclonal antibodies is:
a) Trastuzumab
b) Rituximab
c) OKT-3
d) All of the above

36. Class of OKT-3 is:
a) Immunosuppressive agents
b) Monoclonal antibodies
c) Interferons
d) Immunoglobulins

37. Half-life of OKT-3 is:
a) 18-24 hours
b) 25-35 minutes
c) 4 - 16 hours
d) 21 days

38. The indication for interferon gamma administration is:
a) Idiopathic nephrotic syndrome
b) Hepatitis C virus infection
c) Chronic granulomatous disease
d) Hairy cell leukemia

39. The side effect of interferon gamma is:
a) Hypertension
b) Pulmonary edema
c) Nephrotoxicity
d) Fatigue

40. Half-life of interferon gamma is:
a) 21 days
b) 19 hours
c) 4 - 16 hours
d) 25-35 minutes

41. Half-life of interferon alpha is:
a) 18-24 hours
b) 4-16 hours
c) 25-35 minutes
d) 21 days

42. The indication for interferon alpha administration is:
a) Hepatitis C virus infection
b) Kaposi's sarcoma
c) Condyloma acuminatum
d) All of the above

43. Indication for interferon alpha administration is:
a) Autoimmune diseases
b) Rheumatoid arthritis
c) Organ transplantation
d) Hepatitis C virus infection

44. Indication for interferon alpha administration is:
a) Prophylaxis of sensitization by Rh antigen
b) Rheumatoid arthritis
c) Kaposi's sarcoma
d) Chronic granulomatous disease

45. Class of tacrolimus (FK-506) is:
a) Immunoglobulins
b) Immunosuppressive agents
c) Interferons
d) Monoclonal antibodies

46. Mechanism of action of tacrolimus (FK-506) is:
a) Inhibits CD3 receptor
b) Complement-mediated cytolysis of T lymphocytes
c) Substitution for patient's defiecient immunoglobulins
d) Inhibits calcineurin

47. Immunomodulating agent is:
a) Sirolimus (rapamycin)
b) Levamisole
c) Tacrolimus (FK 506)
d) All of the above

48. Immunomodulating agents are the following EXEPT:
a) Cytokines
b) Levamosole
c) BCG (Bacille Calmette-Guérin)
d) Tacrolimus (FK-506)

49. Mechanism of action of levamisole is:
a) Inhibits CD3 receptor
b) Complement-mediated cytolysis of T lymphocytes
c) Substitution for patient's defiecient immunoglobulins
d) Increase the number of T-cells

Answer Key

01-A,02-A,03-B,04-D,05-A,06-B,07-B,08-D,09-D,10-B,11-D,12-B,13-A,14-A,15-D,16-B,17-C,18-A,19-D,20-D,21-B,22-C,23-D,24-A,25-C,26-D,27-D,28-D,29-D,30-D,31-D,32-B,33-C,34-C,35-D,36-B,37-A,38-D,39-D,40-D,41-B,42-D,43-D,44-C,45-B,46-D,47-B,48-D,49-D

33. Vitamins, Vitamin-like Compounds, Antivitamins, Enzymes & Antienzymes

1.Vitamins are:
a) Inorganic nutrients needed in small quantities in the body
b) Organic substances needed in very large quantities in the body
c) Any of various fat-soluble or water-soluble organic substances essential in minute amounts for normalgrowth and activity of the body and obtained naturally from plant and animal foods
d) Products of endocrine gland secretion

2. Vitamin-like compounds are:
a) A number of compounds, whose nutritional requirements exist at specific periods of development, particularly neonatal development, and periods of rapid growth
b) Inorganic nutrients needed in small quantities in body
c) Organic substances needed in very large quantities in body
d) Products of endocrine gland secretion

3. Antivitamins are:
a) Any of various fat-soluble or water-soluble organic substances essential in minute amounts for normal growth and activity of the body and obtained naturally from plant and animal foods
b) Substances that prevent vitamins from exerting their typical metabolic effects
c) Any of numerous proteins or conjugated proteins produced by living organisms and functioning as specialized catalysts for biochemical reactions
d) Nonprotein organic substances that usually contain a vitamin or mineral and combine with a specific apoenzyme to form an active enzyme system

4. Coenzymes are:
a) Any of various fat-soluble or water-soluble organic substances essential in minute amounts for normal growth and activity of the body and obtained nayurally from plant and animal foods
b) Substances that prevent vitamins from exerting their typical metabolic effects
c) Any of numerous proteins or conjugated proteins produced by living organisms and functioning as specialized catalysts for biochemical reactions

d) Nonprotein organic substances that usually contain a vitamin or mineral and combines with a specific apoenzyme to form an active enzyme system

5. Antienzymes are:
a) Agents, especially an inhibitory enzymes or an antibodies to enzymes, that retard, inhibit, or destroy enzymic activity
b) Substances that prevent vitamins from exerting their typical metabolic effects
c) Any of numerous proteins or conjugated proteins produced by living organisms and functioning as specialized catalysts for biochemical reactions
d) Nonprotein organic substances that usually contain a vitamin or mineral and combines with a specific apoenzyme to form an active enzyme system

6. Select a fat-soluble vitamin:
a) Ascorbic acid
b) Tocopherol
c) Thiamine
d) Riboflavin

7. Select a water-soluble vitamin:
a) Vitamin A
b) Vitamin E
c) Vitamin D
d) Vitamin B$_1$

8. Which of the following vitamins can be also synthesized from a dietary precursor?
a) Vitamin C
b) Vitamin A
c) Vitamin B$_1$
d) Vitamin B$_6$

9. Which of the following vitamins resembles with hormone
a) Vitamin K
b) Vitamin A
c) Vitamin D
d) Vitamin E

10. Beri-beri is caused by the deficiency of:
a) Riboflavin
b) Ascorbic acid
c) Nicotinic acid
d) Thiamine

11. Beri-beri is
a) Disease caused by a deficiency of thiamine, endemic in eastern and southarn Asia, and characterized byneurological symptoms, cardiovascular abnormalities, and edema. It is also called endemic neuritis
b) Inflammation at the corners of the mouth caused by a deficiency of riboflavin, associated with a wrinkled or fissured epithelium that does not involve the mucosa
c) A disorder of the lips often due to riboflavin deficiency and other B-complex vitamin deficiencies and characterized by fissures, especially in the corners of the mouth
d) All of the above

12. Deficiency symptom of riboflavin is:
a) Cheilitis – inflammation of the lips or of a lip, with redness and the production of fissures radiating from the angles of the mouth
b) Cheilosis – a disorder of the lips characterized by fissures, especially in the corners of the mouth
c) Angular stomatitis, associated with a wrinkled or fissured epithelium that does not involve the mucosa
d) All of the above

13. All of the following statements concerning vitamin A functions are true EXCEPT:
a) Transmission of light stimuli to the brain, via combination with a specific protein, opsin, to form a visual pigment,rhodopsin, in the retina of the eye
b) Regulation of cell growth and differentiation in epithelium, connective tissues (including bone and cartilage) and hematopoietic tissues by retinoic acid, a highly bioactive metabolite of retinol
c) Retinoic acid is especially important during embryogenesis
d) Acts as a hormone involved in regulation of calcium and phosphorus homeostasis

14. Deficiency symptom of vitamin A is:
a) Night blindness – lessened ability to see in dim light
b) Xerophthalmia and keratomalacia
c) Various epithelial tissue defects, leading to decreased resistance to infective diseases, male and female infertility
d) All of the above

15. Xerophthalmia is:
a) Extreme dryness of the conjunctiva resulting from a disease localized in the eye or from systemic deficiency of vitamin A

b) A condition, usually in children with vitamin A deficiency, characterized by softening and subsequent ulceration and perforation of the cornea

c) A condition of the eyes in which vision is normal in daylight or other strong light but is abnormally weak or completely lost at night or in dim light and that results from vitamin A deficiency

d) All of the above

16. Keratomalacia is:

a) Extreme dryness of the conjunctiva resulting from a disease localized in the eye or from systemic deficiency of vitamin

b) A condition, usually in children with vitamin A deficiency, characterized by softening and subsequent ulceration and perforation of the cornea

c) A visual defect marked by the inability to see as clearly in bright light as in dim light

d) All of the above

17. Night blindness (Hemeralopia, Nyctalopia) is

a) Extreme dryness of the conjunctiva resulting from a disease localized in the eye or from systemic deficiency of vitamin

b) A condition, usually in children with vitamin A deficiency, characterized by softening and subsequent ulceration and perforation of the cornea

c) A condition of the eyes in which vision is normal in daylight or other strong light but is abnormally weak or completely lost at night or in dim light and that results from vitamin A deficiency

d) All of the above

18. All of the following statements concerning vitamin E functions are true, EXCEPT:

a) An extremely important antioxidant, which protects cell membrane lipids from peroxidation by breaking the chain reaction of free radical formation to which polyunsaturated fatty acids are particularly vulnerable

b) Antisterility and antiabortion factor

c) Specifically required for synthesis of prothrombin and several other clotting factors

d) An essential for oxidative processes regulation

19. Which of the following statements concerning vitamin B1 functions are true:

a) An extremely important antioxidant, which protects cell membrane lipids from peroxidation by breaking the chain reaction of free radical formation to which polyunsaturated fatty acids are particularly vulnerable

b) An essential coenzyme for oxidative decarboxylate of alpha-keto acids, most important being conversion of pyruvate to acetyl coenzyme A

c) Specifically required for synthesis of prothrombin and several other clotting factors

d) Essential constituent of the flavoproteins, flavin mononucleotide (FMN) and flavin adenine dinucleotide (FAD)

20. All of the following statements concerning vitamin B2 functions are true EXCEPT:

a) Essential constituent of flavoproteins, flavin mononucleotide (FMN) and flavin adenine dinucleotide (FAD)

b) Plays key roles in hydrogen transfer reactions associated with glycolysis, TCA cycle and oxidative phosphorylation

c) An essential coenzyme for oxidative decarboxylate of alpha-keto acids, most important being conversion of pyruvate to acetyl coenzyme A

d) Deficiency symptoms are cheilitis, cheilosis and angular stomatitis

21. Which of the following statements concerning vitamin PP (B3, niacin) functions are true:

a) Active group of the coenzymes nicotinamide-adenine dinucleotide (NAD) and nicotinamide-adenine phosphate (NADP)

b) An essential coenzyme for oxidative decarboxylate of alpha-keto acids, most important being conversion of pyruvate to acetyl coenzyme A

c) Specifically required for synthesis of prothrombin and several other clotting factors

d) Essential constituent of flavoproteins, flavin mononucleotide (FMN) and flavin adenine dinucleotide (FAD)

22. Which of the following statements concerning pyridoxine (vitamin B6) functions are true:

a) Active functional form is pyridoxal phosphate, which is an essential coenzyme for transamination and decarboxylation of amino acids in more than 50 different enzyme systems

b) Active group of the coenzymes nicotinamide-adenine dinucleotide (NAD) and nicotinamide-adenine phosphate(NADP)

c) Essential constituent of flavoproteins, flavin mononucleotide (FMN) and flavin adenine dinucleotide (FAD)

d) An extremely important antioxidant, which protects cell membrane lipids from peroxidation by breaking the chainreaction of free radical formation to which polyunsaturated fatty acids are particularly vulnerable

23. Which of the following statements concerning pantothinic acid functions are true:
a) Active functional form is pyridoxal phosphate, which is an essential coenzyme for transamination and decarboxylation of amino acids in more than 50 different enzyme systems
b) Essential constituent of coenzyme A, the important coenzyme for acyl transfer in the TCA cycle and de novo fatty acid synthesis
c) An extremely important antioxidant, which protects cell membrane lipids from peroxidation by breaking the chainreaction of free radical formation to which polyunsaturated fatty acids are particularly vulnerable
d) Coenzyme for several reactions involving CO_2fixation into various compounds e.g. acetyl CoA to malonyl CoA (acetylCoA carboxylase) – initial step in denovo fatty acid synthesis; propionyl CoA to methylmalonyl CoA (propionyl CoAcarboxylase), pyruvate to oxaloacetate (pyruvate carboxylase)

24. Which of the following statements concerning biotin functions are true:
a) Active functional form is pyridoxal phosphate, which is an essential coenzyme for transamination and decarboxylation of amino acids in more than 50 different enzyme systems
b) Essential constituent of coenzyme A, the important coenzyme for acyl transfer in the TCA cycle and de novo fatty acid synthesis
c) An extremely important antioxidant, which protects cell membrane lipids from peroxidation by breaking the chain reaction of free radical formation to which polyunsaturated fatty acids are particularly vulnerable
d) Coenzyme for several reactions involving CO_2 fixation into various compounds e.g. acetyl CoA to malonyl CoA (acetyl CoA carboxylase) – initial step in denovo fatty acid synthesis; propionyl CoA to methylmalonyl CoA (propionyl CoAcarboxylase), pyruvate to oxaloacetate (pyruvate carboxylase)

25. Which of the following statements concerning vitamin B12 (cyanocobalamin) functions are true:
a) Active functional form is pyridoxal phosphate, which is an essential coenzyme for transamination and decarboxylation of amino acids in more than 50 different enzyme systems
b) Essential constituent of coenzyme A, the important coenzyme for acyl transfer in the TCA cycle and de novo fatty acid synthesis
c) Coenzyme for numerous metabolic reaction, including transformation of methylamlonyl CoA to succinyl CoA in the metabolism of propionate; DNA synthesis (acts in concert with folic acid); transmethylation e.g. methionine synthesis from homocysteine

d) An extremely important antioxidant, which protects cell membrane lipids from peroxidation by breaking the chain reaction of free radical formation to which polyunsaturated fatty acids are particularly vulnerable

26. Which of the following statements concerning folic acid (folacin) functions are true:

a) Active functional form is pyridoxal phosphate, which is an essential coenzyme for transamination and decarboxylationof amino acids in more than 50 different enzyme systems

b) Essential constituent of coenzyme A, the important coenzyme for acyl transfer in the TCA cycle and de novo fatty acid synthesis

c) Carrier of one-carbon (e.g. methyl) groups that are added to, or removed from, metabolites such as histidine, serine, methionine, and purines

d) An extremely important antioxidant, which protects cell membrane lipids from peroxidation by breaking the chain reaction of free radical formation to which polyunsaturated fatty acids are particularly vulnerable

27. Which of the following statements concerning vitamin C functions are true:

a) Active functional form is pyridoxal phosphate, which is an essential coenzyme for transamination and decarboxylation of amino acids in more than 50 different enzyme systems

b) Essential constituent of coenzyme A, the important coenzyme for acyl transfer in the TCA cycle and de novo fatty acid synthesis

c) Carrier of one-carbon (e.g. methyl) groups that are added to, or removed from, metabolites such as histidine, serine, methionine, and purines

d) Has antioxidant properties and is required for various hydroxylation reactions e.g. proline to hydroxypoline for collagen synthesis

28. Dermatitis, diarrhoea and dementia are characteristics of:
a) Dry beriberi
b) Pyridoxine deficiency
c) Scurvy
d) Pellagra

29. Pellagra is:
a) A disease caused by a deficiency of niacin in the diet and characterized by skin eruptions, digestive and nervous system disturbances, and eventual mental deterioration
b) Inflammation of several nerves at one time caused by a deficiency of thiamin, marked by paralysis, pain, and muscle wasting. Also called multiple neuritis or polyneuritis

c) A severe form of anemia most often affecting elderly adults, caused by a failure of the stomach to absorb vitamin B_{12} and characterized by abnormally large red blood cells, gastrointestinal disturbances, and lesions of the spinal cord. Also called pernicious anemia, malignant anemia

d) All of the above

30. Pernicious anemia is:

a) A severe form of anemia most often affecting elderly adults, caused by a failure failure of the stomach to absorb vitamin B_{12} and characterized by abnormally large red blood cells, gastrointestinal disturbances, and lesions of the spinal cord

b) A form of anemia in which the capacity of the bone marrow to generate red blood cells is defective, caused by a bonemarrow disease or exposure to toxic agents,such as radiation, chemicals, or drugs

c) Anemia characterized by a decrease in the concentration of corpuscular hemoglobin

d) All of the above

31. Rickets is:

a) A deficiency disease resulting from a lack of vitamin D or calcium and from insufficient exposure to sunlight,characterized by defective bone growth and occurring chiefly in children

b) A disease occurring primarily in adults that results from a deficiency in vitamin D or calcium and is characterized by a softening of the bones with accompanying pain and weakness

c) A disease characterized by a decrease in bone mass and density, occurring especially in postmenopausal women,resulting in a predisposition to fractures and bone deformities such as a vertebral collapse

d) All of the above

32. Scurvy is:

a) A disease caused by deficiency of vitamin C and characterized by spongy bleeding gums, bleeding under the skin, and weakness

b) Extreme dryness of the conjunctiva resulting from a disease localized in the eye or from systemic deficiency of vitamin

c) A disease caused by deficiency of niacin in the diet and characterized by skin eruptions, digestive and nervous system disturbances, and eventual mental deterioration

d) All of the above

33. Which of the following vitamins is given along with isoniazide in treatment of tuberculosis?

a) Nicotinic acid

b) Riboflavin
c) Pyridoxine
d) Ascorbic acid

34. Which of the following vitamins is also known as an antisterility factor?
a) Vitamin E
b) Vitamin B_6
c) Vitamin B_1
 d) Vitamin K

35. Mega doses of which vitamin are some time beneficial viral respiratory infections
a) Vitamin C
b) Vitamin A
c) Vitamin K
d) Vitamin PP

36. Which of the following vitamins improves megaloblast anemia but does not protect the neurological manifestations of pernicious anemia?
a) Vitamin B_{12}
b) Vitamin B_C
c) Vitamin PP
d) Vitamin D

37. Loosening of teeth, gingivitis and hemorrhage occur in the deficiency of:
a) Vitamin K
b) Vitamin B_1
c) Vitamin B_6
d) Vitamin C

38. Ingestion of polar bear liver may cause acute poisoning of:
a) Vitamin D
b) Vitamin E
c) Vitamin A
d) Vitamin C

39. Which of the following antivitamins prevent a vitamin B6 from exerting its typical metabolic effects?
a) Isoniazide
b) Ethanol
c) Carbamazepine
d) All of the above

40. Which of the following antivitamins prevent a vitamin A from exerting its typical metabolic effects?
a) Lipooxidase
b) Oral contraceptives
c) Antibiotics
d) All of the above

41. Which of the following antivitamins prevent a vitamin K from exerting its typical metabolic effects?
a) Cholestiramine
b) Coumarins
c) Antibiotics
d) All of the above

42. Which of the following coenzymes is of vitamin origin?
a) Riboxine
b) Coenzyme Q_{10}
c) Piridixal-5-phosphate
d) Lipoic acid

43. Which of the following coenzymes is not of vitamin origin?
a) Coenzyme Q_{10}
b) Magnesium
c) Carnitine
d) All of the above

44. These substances are vitamin-like compounds, EXCEPT:
a) Choline
b) Vitamin PP
c) Vitamin U (methylmethioninesulfonil chloride)
d) Orotate acid

45. Which of the following substances is a vitamin-like compound?
a) Ascorbic acid
b) Taurine
c) Thiamine
d) Riboflavin

46. Which of the following antienzymes is a proteolysis inhibitor?
a) Contrical
b) Sulbactam

c) Aminocaproic acid

d) Disulfiram

47. Which of the following antienzymes is a beta-lactamase inhibitor?

a) Clavulanic acid

b) Sulbactam

c) Tazobactam

d) All of the above

48. Which of the following antienzymes is a fibrinolysis inhibitor?

a) Clavulanic acid

b) Sulbactam

c) Aminocaproic acid

d) Disulfiram

49. Which of the following antienzymes is an aldehyde dehydrogenase inhibitor?

a) Tazobactam

b) Sulbactam

c) Aminocaproic acid

d) Disulfiram

50. Which of the following antienzymes is a cholinesterase inhibitor?

a) Physostigmine

b) Selegiline

c) Aminocaproic acid

d) Disulfiram

51. Which of the following antienzymes is a monoamine oxidase (MAO) inhibitor:

a) Physostigmine

b) Selegiline

c) Acetazolamide

d) Disulfiram

52. Which of the following antienzymes is a carbonic anhydrase inhibitor:

a) Physostigmine

b) Selegiline

c) Aminocaproic acid

d) Acetazolamide

53. Which of the following antienzymes is a xantine oxidase inhibitor?

a) Physostigmine
b) Allopurinol
c) Aminocaproic acid
d) Acetazolamide

54. Which of the following antienzymes is an aromatase inhibitor used in cancer therapy?

a) Physostigmine
b) Allopurinol
c) Aminocaproic acid
d) Aminoglutethimide

55. Which of the following enzymes improves GIT functions (replacement therapy):

a) Pepsin
b) Urokinase
c) L-asparaginase
d) Lydaze

56. Which of the following enzymes has fibrinolytic activity?

a) Pepsin
b) Urokinase
c) L-asparaginase
d) Lydaze

57. Which of the following enzymes is used in cancer therapy?

a) Pepsin
b) Urokinase
c) L-asparaginase
d) Lydaze

Answer Key

01-C,02-A,03-B,04-D,05-A,06-B,07-D,08-B,09-C,10-D,11-A,12-D,13-D,14-D,15-A,16-B,17-C,18-C,19-B,20-C,21-A,22-A,23-B,24-D,25-C,26-C,27-D,28-D,29-A,30-A,31-A,32-A,33-C,34-A,35-A,36-A,37-D,38-C,39-D,40-A,41-D,42-C,43-D,44-B,45-B,46-A,47-D,48-D,49-D,50-A,51-B,5-D,53-B,54-D,55-A,56-B,57-C

34. Antihyperlipidemic Drugs & Drugs Used In the Treatment of Gout

1. Lipoprotein is:
a) A conjugated protein having a lipid component; the principal means for transporting lipids in the blood
b) Any of various fat-soluble or water-soluble organic substances essential in minute amounts for normal growth and activity of the body and obtained naturally from plant and animal foods
c) Product of endocrine gland secretion
d) Mediators of inflammatory process

2. Very low density lipoprotein (VLDL) is:
a) A lipoprotein containing a very large proportion of lipids to protein and carrying most cholesterol from the liver to the tissues
b) A lipoprotein that contains relatively high amounts of cholesterol and is associated with an increased risk of atherosclerosis and coronary artery disease. it is also called beta-lipoprotein
c) A lipoprotein that contains relatively small amounts of cholesterol and triglycerides and is associated with a decreased risk of atherosclerosis and coronary artery disease. It is also called alpha-lipoprotein
d) Large lipoprotein particle that is created by the absorptive cells of the small intestine. It transports lipids to adipose tissue where they are broken down by lipoprotein lipase

3. Low-density lipoprotein (LDL) is:
a) A lipoprotein that contains relatively high amounts of cholesterol and is associated with an increased risk of atherosclerosis and coronary artery disease. it is also called beta-lipoprotein
b) A lipoprotein that contains relatively small amounts of cholesterol and triglycerides and is associated with a decreasedrisk of atherosclerosis and coronary artery disease. It is also called alpha-lipoprotein
c) A lipoprotein containing a very large proportion of lipids to protein and carrying most cholesterol from the liver to thetissues
d) Large lipoprotein particle that is created by the absorptive cells of the small intestine. It transports lipids to adipose tissue where they are broken down by lipoprotein lipase

4. High-density lipoprotein (HDL) is:

a) A lipoprotein that contains relatively small amounts of cholesterol and triglycerides and is associated with a decreased risk of atherosclerosis and coronary artery disease. It is also called alpha-lipoprotein

b) A lipoprotein containing a very large proportion of lipids to protein and carrying most cholesterol from the liver to the tissues

c) A lipoprotein that contains relatively high amounts of cholesterol and is associated with an increased risk ofatherosclerosis and coronary artery disease. It is also called beta-lipoprotein

d) Large lipoprotein particle that is created by the absorptive cells of the small intestine. It transports lipids to adipose tissue where they are broken down by lipoprotein lipase

5. Chylomicron is:

a) A lipoprotein that contains relatively small amounts of cholesterol and triglycerides and is associated with a decreasedrisk of atherosclerosis and coronary artery disease. It is also called alpha-lipoprotein

b) A lipoprotein containing a very large proportion of lipids to protein and carrying most cholesterol from the liver to thetissues

c) A lipoprotein that contains relatively high amounts of cholesterol and is associated with an increased risk ofatherosclerosis and coronary artery disease. It is also called beta-lipoprotein

d) Large lipoprotein particle that is created by the absorptive cells of the small small intestine. It transports lipids to adipose tissue where they are broken down by lipoprotein lipase

6. All of the following statements concerning cholestyramine (Questran) are true, EXCEPT:

a) It would not be a good choice for treating patients with familial hypertriglyceridemia (type IV)

b) It is not well tolerated by patients

c) It works by directly binding cholesterol in the blood

d) It is an effective drug for treatment of types IIa and IIb hyperlipidemia

7. All of the following statements concerning drugs which inhibit cholesterol synthesis are true, EXCEPT:

a) They work in part by increasing the rate of LDL clearance from the plasma

b) They are the most effective single agents for lowering LDL-cholesterol

c) When used with a bile-acid binding resin, they can lower LDL-cholesterol by 50% or more

d) No special monitoring is required in patients receiving one of them

8. All of the following statements concerning nicotinic acid (Niacin) are true, EXCEPT:

a) It reduces the rate of synthesis of VLDL

b) Sustained-release preparations of this drug are largely free of side effects

c) Almost all patients taking the traditional dosage form of this drug experience uncomfortable flushing

d) It should not be used with antihypertensives

9. All of the following statements concerning drugs which inhibit cholesterol synthesis are true, EXCEPT:

a) When used alone, they are the most effective agents for lowering LDL cholesterol

b) They are often effective in patients in whom a diet, with or without a bile acid-binding resin or niacin, has failed

c) Lovastatin (Mevacor) plus a resin causes regression of coronary lesions in about one third of treated patients

d) Members of this drug class are generally not as well tolerated as the older bile acid-binding resins

10. All of the following statements concerning drugs which inhibit cholesterol synthesis are true, EXCEPT:

a) These drugs should not be used in pregnant women or children

b) These drugs often cause myopathy if used in combination with cyclosporine (Sandimmune)

c) Failure to discontinue the drug after myopathy has been detected can cause acute renal failure

d) Several of these drugs tend to lengthen the sleep cycle

11. All of the following statements concerning the fibric acid derivatives are true, EXCEPT:

a) Clofibrate (Atromid-S) is the drug of choice for therapy of Type III hyperlipidemia

b) Gemfibrozil (Lopid) increases HDL cholesterol while lowering LDL cholesterol

c) Gemfibrozil (Lopid) has been shown to reduce mortality associated with a heart disease

d) Gemfibrozil (Lopid) is generally well tolerated

12. All of the following statements concerning the bile acid-binding resins are true, EXCEPT:

a) They decrease total cholesterol and LDL

b) They are contraindicated in patients with hypertriglyceridemia

c) When used alone, they do not slow the progression of atherosclerotic lesions

d) They are the drugs of choice for therapy of type II hyperlipidemia when used either alone or in combination with selected agents

13. All of the following statements concerning nicotinic acid (Niacin) are true, EXCEPT:

a) Both triglycerides and LDL cholesterol are reduced by this drug

b) The drug acts by directly decreasing the rate of synthesis of apoproteins

c) Doses higher than 3 gm/day are no longer used because of possible disturbances of hepatic or pancreatic functions

d) Most patients taking this drug experience uncomfortable cutaneous flushing, itching, and/or rashes

14. All of the following statements concerning the general principles of therapy with lipid-lowering drugs are true EXCEPT:

a) Therapy with a lipid-lowering drug should be always accompanied by an appropriate diet

b) A lipid-lowering diet should be discontinued if it fails to decrease the levels of plasma LDL cholesterol by at least 10%

c) Lipid-lowering drugs should only be administered after at least 3 months of prior dietary therapy

d) Some combinations of lipid-lowering drugs are synergistic

15. This drug increases lipoprotein lipase (LPL) activity in adipose tissue:

a) Cholestyramine (Questran)

b) Lovastatin (Mevacor)

c) Nicotinic acid (Niacin)

d) Gemfibrozil (Loprol)

16. This drug both inhibits an enzyme and indirectly enhances clearance of low density lipoproteins (LDL):

a) Cholestyramine (Questran)

b) Lovastatin (Mevacor)

c) Nicotinic acid (niacin)

d) Probucol (Lorelco)

17. This drug binds bile acids in the GI tract:

a) Cholestyramine (Questran)

b) Nicotinic acid (niacin)

c) Gemfibrozil (Loprol)

d) Probucol (Lorelco)

18. This drug may block oxidation of low density lipoproteins (LDL):
a) Lovastatin (Mevacor)
b) Nicotinic acid (niacin)
c) Gemfibrozil (Loprol)
d) Probucol (Lorelco)

19. This drug weakly stimulates synthesis of very low density lipoproteins (VLDL):
a) Cholestyramine (Questran)
b) Lovastatin (Mevacor)
c) Gemfibrozil (Loprol)
d) Probucol (Lorelco)

20. Flushing caused by this drug can be reduced by taking it after meals and/or by pretreatment with aspirin:
a) Lovastatin (Mevacor)
b) Nicotinic acid (niacin)
c) Gemfibrozil (Loprol)
d) Probucol (Lorelco)

21. This drug can cause muscle damage, especially when used with any of several drugs including erythromycin:
a) Cholestyramine (Questran)
b) Lovastatin (Mevacor)
c) Gemfibrozil (Loprol)
d) Probucol (Lorelco)

22. This drug decreases blood levels of high density lipoproteins (HDL):
a) Lovastatin (Mevacor)
b) Nicotinic acid (niacin)
c) Gemfibrozil (Loprol)
d) Probucol (Lorelco)

23. This fibric acid derivative increases blood levels of high density lipoproteins (HDL):
a) Cholestyramine (Questran)
b) Lovastatin (Mevacor)
c) Gemfibrozil (Loprol)
d) Probucol (Lorelco)

24. Which of the following drugs is an uricosuric agent:
a) Allopurinol
b) Sulfinpyrazone
c) Colchicine
d) Indomethacin

25. Uricosuric drugs are the following, EXCEPT:
a) Probenecid
b) Sulfinpyrazone
c) Colchicine
d) Aspirin (at high dosages)

26. Which of the following drugs used in the treatment of gout acts by preventing the migration of granulocytes:
a) Allopurinol
b) Sulfinpyrazone
c) Colchicine
d) Indomethacin

27. Which of the following drugs used in the treatment of gout has as its primary effect the reduction of uric acid synthesis
a) Allopurinol
b) Sulfinpyrazone
c) Colchicine
d) Indomethacin

28. Characteristics of probenecid include all of the following, EXCEPT:
a) It promotes the renal tubular secretion of penicillin
b) It is useful in the treatment of gout
c) At appropriate doses, it promotes the excretion of uric acid
d) The metabolic products of probenecid are uricosuric

Answer Key

01-A,02-A,03,A,04-A,05-D,06-C,07-D,08-B,09-D,10-D,11-A,12-C,13-B,14-B,15-D,16-B,17-A,18-D,19-A,20-B,21-B,2-D,23-C,24-B,25-C,26-C,27-A,28-A

35. Agents That Affect Bone Mineral Homeostasis

1. Action of the parathyroid hormone is:
a) Increased calcium and phosphate absorption in intestine (by increased 1,25-dihydroxyvitamin D_3production)
b) Decreased calcium excretion and increased phosphate excretion in kidneys
c) In bone, calcium and phosphate resorption increased by high doses. Low doses may increase bone formation.
d) All of the above

2. The following statements about the parathyroid hormone are true, EXCEPT:
a) The parathyroid hormone (PTH) is a single-chain peptide hormone composed of 84 amino acids
b) The parathyroid hormone increases calcium and phosphate absorption in intestine (by increased 1,25-dihydroxyvitamin D_3production)
c) The parathyroid hormone increases serum calcium and decreases serum phosphate
d) The parathyroid hormone increases calcium excretion and decreases phosphate excretion in kidneys

3. Which of the following statements about calcitonin is true:
a) Calcitonin secreted by parafollicular cells of the mammalian thyroid is a single-chain peptide hormone with 32 amino acids
b) Effects of calcitonin are to lower serum calcium and phosphate by acting on bones and kidneys.
c) Calcitonin inhibits osteoclastic bone resorption.
d) All of the above

4. Mechanism of action of calcitonin is:
a) Inhibits hydroxyapatite crystal formation, aggregation, and dissolution
b) Raises intracellular cAMP in osteoclasts
c) Activates bone resorption
d) Inhibits macrophages

5. Indications for calcitonin administration are the following, EXCEPT:
a) Hypercalcemia
b) Paget's disease
c) Hypophosphatemia
d) Osteoporosis

6. Side effect of calcitonin is:
a) Hypercalcemia
b) Metastatic calcifications
c) Tetany
d) GI toxicity

7. Side effect of calcitonin is:
a) Pruritus
b) Hypotension
c) Fractures
d) Hypocalcemia

8. Glucocorticoid hormones alter bone mineral homeostasis:
a) By antagonizing vitamin D-stimulated intestinal calcium transport
b) By stimulating renal calcium excretion
c) By increasing parathyroid hormone stimulated bone resorption
d) By all of the above

9. Action of vitamin D3 is:
a) Increased calcium and phosphate absorption by 1,25-dihydroxyvitamin D_3
b) Calcium and phosphate excretion may be decreased by 25-hydroxyvitamin D_3 and 1,25-dihydroxyvitamin D_3
c) Increased calcium and phosphate resorption by 1,25-dihydroxyvitamin D_3; bone formation may be increased by 25,24-dihydroxyvitamin D_3
d) All of the above

10. Route of administration of vitamin D3 is:
a) Subcutaneous
b) Oral
c) Intravenous
d) Intranasal

10. Side effect of vitamin D3 is:
a) Defective bone mineralization
b) Metastatic calcifications
c) Hepatic toxicity
d) Nephrolithiasis

11. Indication of vitamin D3 is:
a) Hypercalcemia
b) Paget's disease
c) Hypophosphatemia
d) Osteomalacia

12. Route of administration of 25-hydroxyvitamin D3 (calcifediol) is:
a) Oral
b) Subcutaneous
c) Intravenous
d) Intranasal

13. Indication for 25-hydroxyvitamin D3 (calcifediol) administration is:
a) Primary hyperparathyroidism
b) Rickets
c) Hypercalcemia
d) Failure of vitamin D formation in skin

14. Side effect of 25-hydroxyvitamin D3 (calcifediol) is:
a) Hypercalcemia
b) Pruritus
c) GI toxicity
d) All of the above

15. Indications for 1,25-dihydroxyvitamin D3 (calcitriol) administration are the following, EXCEPT:
a) Hypocalcemia in chronic renal failure
b) Vitamin D-dependent rickets
c) Malabsorption of vitamin D from intestine
d) Elevated skeletal turnover

16. Indication for 1,25-dihydroxyvitamin D3 (calcitriol) administration is:
a) Vitamin D resistance
b) Elevated skeletal turnover
c) Hypercalcemia of malignancy
d) Hypophosphatemia

17. The following statement refers to 1,25-dihydroxyvitamin D3 (calcitriol):
a) When rapidity of action is required, 1,25-dihydroxyvitamin D_3(calcitriol), 0.25-1 µg daily, is the vitamin D metabolite of
choice, since it is capable of raising serum calcium within 24-48 hours

b) Calcitriol also raises serum phosphate, though this action is usually not observed early in treatment

c) Undergoes enterohepatic circulation

d) All of the above

18. Which of the following statements refers to 1,25-dihydroxyvitamin D3 (calcitriol):

a) The combined effect of calcitriol and all other vitamin D metabolites and analogs on both calcium and phosphate makes careful monitoring of the level of these minerals especially important to avoid ectopiccalcification

b) Does not undergo enterohepatic circulation

c) Toxic to osteoclasts

d) Bioavailability increases with the administered dose

19. Route of administration of 1,25-dihydroxyvitamin D3 (calcitriol) is:

a) Subcutaneous

b) Intravenous

c) Intranasal

d) Oral

20. Commercially available analogs of 1,25-dihydroxyvitamin D3 (calcitriol) are:

a) Doxercalciferol (Hectoral)

b) Paricalcitol (Zemplar)

c) All of the above

d) None of the above

21. Side effect of dihydrotachysterol is:

a) Hepatic toxicity

b) General malaise

c) Lymphocytopenia

d) Hypertension

22. Route of administration of dihydrotachysterol is:

a) Intravenous

b) Subcutaneous

c) Oral

d) Intranasal

23. Which of the following statements refers to cholecalciferol:

a) Frequent monitoring of both calcium and phosphorus serum levels is necessary in case of intravenous administration

b) Has potent anti-osteoclast activity – mechanism unknown

c) Can usually lower serum calcium levels in 48 hours

d) Mechanism of action: 1. Genomic effects 2. Cytoplasmic effects

24. Indication for cholecalciferol administration is:

a) Hypercalcemia

b) Parathyroid hormone deficiency

c) Primary hyperparathyroidism

d) Malabsorption of vitamin D from intestine

25. Route of administration of cholecalciferol is:

a) Subcutaneous

b) Intranasal

c) Intravenous

d) Oral

26. The unwanted effect of cholecalciferol is:

a) Defective bone mineralization

b) Lymphocytopenia

c) CNS toxicity

d) Metastatic calcifications

27. The unwanted effect of dihydrotachysterol is:

a) Tetany

b) Anorexia

c) CNS toxicity

d) Lymphocytopenia

28. Indication for dihydrotachysterol administration is:

a) Parathyroid hormone resistance

b) Paget's disease

c) Increased osteolysis

d) Hypophosphatemia

29. Conditions associated with hypophosphatemia include:

a) Primary hyperparathyroidism

b) Vitamin D deficiency

c) Idiopathic hypercalciuria

d) All of the above.

30. Recommended phosphorus daily allowance is:
a) 900-1200 mg
b) 600-900 g
c) 25 g
d) 1.5-4 mg

31. Interactions with other drugs of phosphorus is:
a) Amiloride: decrease renal excretion
b) Glucocorticoids: decrease absorption
c) Loop diuretics: increase renal excretion
d) Calcitonin: increases renal excretion

32. Indication for pamidronate administration is:
a) Failure of vitamin D formation in skin
b) Hypoparathyroidism
c) Elevated skeletal turnover
d) Hypercalcemia

33. Route of administration of pamidronate is:
a) Oral
b) Subcutaneous
c) Intranasal
d) Intravenous

34. Correct statements about pamidronate include all of the following, EXCEPT:
a) Because it causes gastric irritation, pamidronate is not available as an oral preparation
b) Skeletal half-life is 24 h
c) Fever and lymphocytopenia are reversible
d) Can be irritable to the esophagus if not washed promptly to the stomach

35. Route of administration of alendronate is:
a) Intravenous
b) Subcutaneous
c) Oral
d) Intranasal

36. Indications of alendronate are the following, EXCEPT:
a) Hypoparathyroidism
b) Glucocorticoid-induced osteoporosis
c) Paget's disease
d) Syndromes of ectopic calcification

37. Indication for etidronate administration is:
a) Malabsorption of vitamin D from intestine
b) Paget's disease
c) Vitamin D deficiency in a diet
d) Hypercalciuria

38. Indications for etidronate administration are the following, EXEPT:
a) Paget's disease
b) Osteoporosis
c) Hypophosphatemia
d) Hypercalcemia

39. Which of the following statements refers to etidronate:
a) Reduces osteoclast activity without significantly affecting osteoblasts; useful in treatment of Paget's disease
b) Serum phosphorus concentrations should be monitored at least daily in case of oral administration
c) 2nd generation biphosphonate (amino-biphosphonate)
d) Bioavailability increases with the administered dose

40. Correct statements about etidronate include all of the following, EXCEPT:
a) Skeletal half-life is hundreds of days
b) Bioavailability increases with the administered dose
c) 2nd generation biphosphonate (amino-biphosphonate)
d) 1st generation biphosphonate.

41. Unwanted effect of etidronate is:
a) Anorexia
b) Defective bone mineralization
c) Hypercalcemia
d) Cardiac arrhythmias

42. The major causes of hypocalcemia in the adult are:
a) Hypoparathyroidism
b) Vitamin D deficiency
c) Renal failure and malabsorption
d) All of the above

43. The major causes of hypercalcemia in the adult are the following, EXCEPT :
a) Hyperparathyroidism
b) Cancer with or without bone metastases

c) Renal failure and malabsorption
d) Hypervitaminosis D

44. Which of the following statements refers to calcium:
a) Recommended Ca daily allowance for males: 1. 1-10 years: 800 mg 2. 11-18 years: 1200 mg 3. 19-50 years: 1000 mg 4. > 51 years: 1000 mg
b) Ca chloride is very irritating and can cause necrosis if extravasated
c) In achlorhydric patients calcium carbonate should be given with meals to increase absorption or patient switched to calcium citrate, which is somewhat better absorbed
d) All of the above

45. Indication for calcium administration is:
a) Failure of formation of vitamin D in skin
b) Malabsorption of vitamin D from intestine
c) Hypercalcemia of malignancy
d) Vitamin D deficiency

46. Which of the calcium preparations is the most preferable for IV injection
a) Calcium gluceptate (0.9 meq calcium/mL)
b) Calcium gluconate (0.45 meq calcium/mL)
c) Calcium chloride (0.68-1.36 meq calcium/mL)
d) All of the above

47. Which of the oral calcium preparations is often the preparation of choice:
a) Calcium carbonate (40% calcium)
b) Calcium lactate (13% calcium)
c) Calcium phosphate (25% calcium)
d) Calcium citrate (17% calcium)

48. Interactions with other drugs of calcium is:
a) Ethanol: decreases absorption
b) Loop diuretics: increase renal excretion
c) Glucocorticoids: stimulate renal excretion
d) All of the above

49. Correct statements about magnesium include all of the following, EXCEPT:
a) Magnesium is mainly an intracellular cation, and is the fourth most abundant cation in the body
b) The recommended dietary amounts of magnesium have been set at 6 mg/kg day (350-400 mg)

c) The most common specific causes encountered in clinical practice are: diet, alcoholism (drinking), diarrhea and malabsorption, diabetes mellitus, diuretics, and drugs such as aminoglycosides and amphotericin

d) It is a physiological calcium agonist

50. Recommended magnesium daily allowance is:
a) 350-400 mg
b) 6-9 g
c) 25 g
d) 1.5-4 mg

51. The major causes of hypomagnesaemia are:
a) Insufficient dietary intake, e.g. malnutrition
b) Abnormal gastrointestinal loss, e.g. severe diarrhea or chronic alcoholism
c) Abnormal renal loss, e.g. diabetes mellitus or during therapy with some kind of drugs such as amphotericin B,gentamicin, cisplatin, cardiac glycosides, distal and loop diuretics
d) All of the above

52. Which of the magnesium preparation is the most preferable for I.V. injection
a) Magnesium sulfate
b) Magnesium chloride
c) Magnesium glutamate
d) All of the above

53. Which of the oral magnesium preparations is often the preparation of choice:
a) Magnesium lactate
b) Magnesium oxide
c) MagneB$_6$ (Mg pidolate / Mg lactate + pyridoxine hydrochloride)
d) All of the above.

54. Correct statements about fluoride include all of the following, EXCEPT:
a) Fluoride is effective for the prophylaxis of dental caries
b) Fluoride is accumulated by bone and teeth, where it may stabilize the hydroxyapatite crystal
c) Subjects living in areas with naturally fluoridated water (1-2 ppm) had more dental caries and fewer vertebral compression fractures than subjects living in non-fluoridated water areas

d) Chronic exposure to very high level of fluoride dust in the inspired air results in crippling fluorosis, characterized by thickening of the cortex of long bones and bony exostoses.

55. Recommended fluoride daily allowance is:
a) 1.5-4 mg
b) 600-900 g
c) 25 g
d) 350-400 mg

56. Which of the following statements refers to gallium nitrate:
a) It is approved by the FDA for the management of hypercalcemia of malignancy
b) This drug acts by inhibiting bone resorption
c) Because of potential nephrotoxicity, patients should be well-hydrated and have good renal output before starting the infusion
d) All of the above

57. Which of the following statements refers to plicamycin (formerly mithramycin):
a) Duration of action is usually several days
b) Mechanism of cytotoxic action appears to involve its binding to DNA, possibly through an antibiotic-Mg^{2+} complex.
c) The drug causes plasma calcium levels to decrease, apparently through an action on osteoclasts that is independent of its action on tumor cells and useful in hypercalcemia.
d) All of the above.

58. Unwanted effects of plicamycin (formerly mithramycin) are the following, EXEPT:
a) Thrombocytopenia
b) GI toxicity
c) Bleeding disorders
d) Fractures

59. Unwanted effect of plicamycin (formerly mithramycin) is:
a) Diarrhea
b) Myelosuppression
c) Nephrolithiasis
d) Metastatic calcifications

60. Indication for plicamycin (formerly mithramycin) administration is:
a) Testicular cancers refractory to standard treatment
b) Paget's disease
c) Hypercalcemia of malignancy
d) All of the above

61. Route of administration of plicamycin is:
a) Intravenous
b) Subcutaneous
c) Intranasal
d) Oral

Answer Key

01-D,02-D,03-D,04-B,05-C,06-C,07-B,08-D,09-D,10-B,11-C,12-A,13-D,14-D,15-D,16-D,17-D,18-A,19-D,20-C,21-D,22-C,23-D,24-D,25-D,26-C,27-C,28-D,29-D,30-A,31-D,32-D,33-D,34-B,35-C,36-A,37-B,38-C,39-D,40-C,41-B,42-D,43-C,44-D,45-D,46-B,47-A,48-D,49-A,48-D,49-D,50-A,51-D,52-B,53-C,54-C,55-A,56-D,57-D,58-D,59-B,60-D,61-A

36. Mineralocorticoid, Mineralocorticoid Antagonists, Diuretics, Plasma Expanders

1. Mineralocorticoid effects cause:
a) Increased catabolism
b) Increased Na retension and K excretion
c) Increased gluconeogenesis
d) Deposition of fat on shoulders, face and abdomen

2. Which of the following synthetic steroids shows predominantly mineralocorticoid action?
a) Hydrocortisone
b) Spironolactone
c) Dexamethasone
d) Fludrocortisone

3. The major mineralocorticoids are the following, EXCEPT:
a) Aldosterone
b) Deoxycorticosterone
c) Fludrocortisone
d) Hydrocortisone

4. Which of the following statements about spironolactone is TRUE?
a) Spironolactone reverses many of the manifestations of aldosteronism
b) Spironilactone is also an androgen antagonist and as such is used in the treatment of hirsutism in wormen
c) Spironolactone is useful as a diuretic
d) All of the above

5. All of the following statements regarding diuretics are true, EXCEPT:
a) Carbonic anhydrase inhibition leads to increased reabsorption of $NaHCO_3$
b) Loop diuretics decrease Na^+ reabsorption at the loop of Henle by competing for the Cl^- site on the $Na^+/K^+/2Cl^-$ cotransporter
c) In general, the potency of a diuretic is determined by where it acts in the renal tubule
d) Hydrochlorothiazide decreases urinary calcium excretion

6. The drug inhibits the ubiquitous enzyme carbonic anhydrase:
a) Acetazolamide (Diamox)
b) Furosemide (Lasix)
c) Hydrochlorothiazide (HydroDiuril)
d) Spironolactone (Aldactone)

7. The drug acts by competitively blocking NaCl cotransporters in the distal tubule:
a) Acetazolamide (Diamox)
b) Furosemide (Lasix)
c) Hydrochlorothiazide (HydroDiuril)
d) Spironolactone (Aldactone)

8. The drug acts at the proximal tubule:
a) Acetazolamide (Diamox)
b) Furosemide (Lasix)
c) Hydrochlorothiazide (HydroDiuril)
d) Spironolactone (Aldactone)

9. The drug acts by competing with aldosterone for its cytosolic receptors:
a) Acetazolamide (Diamox)
b) Furosemide (Lasix)
c) Hydrochlorothiazide (HydroDiuril)
d) Spironolactone (Aldactone)

10. The drug is a potassium-sparing diuretic that blocks Na+ channels in the collecting tubules:
a) Acetazolamide (Diamox)
b) Amiloride (Midamor)
c) Furosemide (Lasix)
d) Hydrochlorothiazide (HydroDiuril)

11. Chronic use of this drug can lead to distal tubular hypertrophy, which may reduce its diuretic effect:
a) Acetazolamide (Diamox)
b) Amiloride (Midamor)
c) Furosemide (Lasix)
d) Hydrochlorothiazide (HydroDiuril)

12. The drug has a steroid-like structure which is responsible for its anti-androgenic effect:
a) Amiloride (Midamor)

b) Furosemide (Lasix)

c) Hydrochlorothiazide (HydroDiuril)

d) Spironolactone (Aldactone)

13. Sustained use of this drug results in increased plasma urate concentrations:

a) Furosemide (Lasix)

b) Acetazolamide (Diamox)

c) Both of the above

d) Neither of the above

14. The drug can be used to treat glaucoma:

a) Furosemide (Lasix)

b) Acetazolamide (Diamox)

c) Both of the above

d) Neither of the above

15. The drug can cause ototoxicity:

a) Furosemide (Lasix)

b) Acetazolamide (Diamox)

c) Both of the above

d) Neither of the above

16. The drug acts only on the lumenal side of renal tubules:

a) Furosemide (Lasix)

b) Acetazolamide (Diamox)

c) Both of the above

d) Neither of the above

17. The drug can promote sodium loss in patients with low (e.g., 40 ml/min) glomerular filtration rates:

a) Furosemide (Lasix)

b) Acetazolamide (Diamox)

c) Both of the above

d) Neither of the above

18. The drug needs aldosterone present in order to be effective:

a) Hydrochlorothiazide (HydroDiuril)

b) Amiloride (Midamor)

c) Both of the above

d) Neither of the above

19. The drug can be used to treat nephrogenic diabetes insipidus:
a) Hydrochlorothiazide (HydroDiuril)
b) Amiloride (Midamor)
c) Both of the above
d) Neither of the above

20. The drug is sometimes part of fixed-dose combinations used to treat essential hypertension:
a) Hydrochlorothiazide (HydroDiuril)
b) Amiloride (Midamor)
c) Both of the above
d) Neither of the above

21. The drug should never be administered to patients taking potassium supplements:
a) Hydrochlorothiazide (HydroDiuril)
b) Amiloride (Midamor)
c) Furosemide (Lasix)
d) Neither of the above

22. The drug decreases calcium excretion in urine:
a) Hydrochlorothiazide (HydroDiuril)
b) Amiloride (Midamor)
c) Furosemide (Lasix)
d) Acetazolamide (Diamox)

23. The drug acts by competitively blocking the Na+/K+/2Cl- cotransporter:
a) Loop diuretics
b) Thiazide diuretics
c) Potassium-sparing diuretics
d) Carbonic anhydrase inhibitors

24. The drug acts at the proximal tubule:
a) Loop diuretics
b) Thiazide diuretics
c) Potassium-sparing diuretics
d) Carbonic anhydrase inhibitors

25. The drug acts in the distal convoluted tubule:
a) Loop diuretics
b) Thiazide diuretics
c) Potassium-sparing diuretics
d) Carbonic anhydrase inhibitors

26. The drug acts in the collecting tubules:
a) Loop diuretics
b) Thiazide diuretics
c) Potassium-sparing diuretics
d) Carbonic anhydrase inhibitors

27. The drug is the most potent diuretic:
a) Loop diuretics
b) Thiazide diuretics
c) Potassium-sparing diuretics
d) Carbonic anhydrase inhibitors

28. The drug acts by competitively blocking the NaCl cotransporter:
a) Loop diuretics
b) Thiazide diuretics
c) Potassium-sparing diuretics
d) Carbonic anhydrase inhibitors

29. The drug inhibits sodium and chloride transport in the cortical thick ascending limb and the early distal tubule:
a) Acetazolamide (Diamox)
b) Furosemide (Lasix)
c) Hydrochlorothiazide (Hydrodiuril)
d) Amiloride (Midamor)

30. The drug can cause ototoxicity:
a) Acetazolamide (Diamox)
b) Furosemide (Lasix)
c) Hydrochlorothiazide (Hydrodiuril)
d) Amiloride (Midamor)

31. The drug blocks the sodium/potassium/chloride cotransporter in the thick ascending loop of Henle:
a) Acetazolamide (Diamox)
b) Furosemide (Lasix)
c) Hydrochlorothiazide (Hydrodiuril)
d) Amiloride (Midamor)

32. The drug is one of the most potent diuretics:
a) Acetazolamide (Diamox)
b) Furosemide (Lasix)
c) Hydrochlorothiazide (Hydrodiuril)
d) Amiloride (Midamor)

33. The drug is usually given in combination with a thiazide diuretic:
a) Acetazolamide (Diamox)
b) Furosemide (Lasix)
c) Hydrochlorothiazide (Hydrodiuril)
d) Amiloride (Midamor)

34. All of the following statements regarding diuretics are true EXCEPT:
a) Furosemide (Lasix) can increase the likelihood of digitalis toxicity
b) Chlorthalidone (Hygroton) can decrease the excretion of lithium
c) Ibuprofen can increase the antihypertensive effect of chlorthalidone
d) Chlorthalidone has a longer duration of action than furosemide

35. The drug is the least potent diuretic:
a) Osmotic diuretics
b) Loop diuretics
c) Thiazide diuretics
d) Potassium-sparing diuretics

36. These agents must be given parenterally because they are not absorbed when given orally:
a) Osmotic diuretics
b) Loop diuretics
c) Thiazide diuretics
d) Potassium-sparing diuretics

37. These drugs may be used in the treatment of recurrent calcium nephrolithiasis:
a) Osmotic diuretics
b) Loop diuretics
c) Thiazide diuretics
d) Potassium-sparing diuretics

38. Furosemide (Lasix) acts at this nephron site:
a) Proximal convoluted tubule
b) Ascending thick limb of the loop of Henle
c) Distal convoluted tubule
d) Collecting duct

39. Metolazone (Mykrox) acts at this nephron site:
a) Proximal convoluted tubule
b) Ascending thick limb of the loop of Henle
c) Distal convoluted tubule
d) Collecting duct

40. Acetazolamide (Diamox) acts at this nephron site:
a) Proximal convoluted tubule
b) Ascending thick limb of the loop of Henle
c) Distal convoluted tubule
d) Collecting duct

41. Spironolactone (Aldactone) acts at this nephron site:
a) Proximal convoluted tubule
b) Ascending thick limb of the loop of Henle
c) Distal convoluted tubule
d) Collecting duct

42. Amiloride (Midamone) acts at this nephron site:
a) Proximal convoluted tubule
b) Ascending thick limb of the loop of Henle
c) Distal convoluted tubule
d) Collecting duct

43. The drug competitively blocks chloride channels and prevents movement of sodium, potassium, and chloride into the renal tubular cells:
a) Furosemide (Lasix)
b) Acetazolamide (Diamox)
c) Triamterene (Dyrenium)
d) Mannitol (Osmitrol)

44. The drug acts by affecting the tubular fluid composition in a non-receptor mediated fashion:
a) Furosemide (Lasix)
b) Acetazolamide (Diamox)
c) Triamterene (Dyrenium)
d) Mannitol (Osmitrol)

45. The drug is a blood substitute having haemodynamical activity:
a) Polyglucinum
b) Haemodesum
c) Sodium chloridum isotonic for injections
d) "Disolum", "Trisolum"

46. This drug is a desintoxicative plasma substitute:
a) Polyglucinum
b) Haemodesum
c) Sodium chloridum isotonic for injections
d) "Disolum", "Trisolum"

47. This drug is a controller of water-salt and acid-basic state:
a) Polyglucinum
b) Haemodesum
c) Glucose isotonic for injections
d) "Disolum", "Trisolum"

Answer Key

01-B,02-D,03-D,04-D,05-A,06-A,07-C,08-A,09-D,10-B,11-C,12-D,13-A,14-B,15-A,16-A,17-A,18-D,19-A,20-C,21-B,22-A,23-A,24-D,25-B,26-C,27-A,28-B,29-C,30-B,31-B,32-B,33-D,34-C,35-D,36-A,37-B,38-B,39-C,40-A,41-D,42-D,43-A,44-D,45-A,46-B,47-D

37. Antibiotics

1.What does the term "antibiotics" mean:
a) Non-organic or synthetic substances that selectively kill or inhibit the growth of other microorganisms
b) Substances produced by some microorganisms and their synthetic analogues that selectively kill or inhibit the growth of another microorganisms
c) Substances produced by some microorganisms and their synthetic analogues that inhibit the growth of organism cells
d) Synthetic analogues of natural substances that kill protozoa and helminthes

2. General principles of anti-infective therapy are:
a) Clinical judgment of microbiological factors
b) Definitive identification of a bacterial infection and the microorganism's susceptibility
c) Optimal route of administration, dose, dosing frequency and duration of treatment
d) All of the above

3. Minimal duration of antibacterial treatment usually is:
a) Not less than 1 day
b) Not less than 5 days
c) Not less than 10-14 days
d) Not less than 3 weeks

4. Rational anti-microbial combination is used to:
a) Provide synergism when microorganisms are not effectively eradicated with a single agent alone
b) Provide broad coverage
c) Prevent the emergence of resistance
d) All of the above

5. Mechanisms of bacterial resistance to anti-microbial agents are the following, EXCEPT:
a) Active transport out of a microorganism or/and hydrolysis of an agent via enzymes produced by a microorganism
b) Enlarged uptake of the drug by a microorganism
c) Modification of a drug's target
d) Reduced uptake by a microorganism

6. All of the following drugs are antibiotics, EXCEPT:
a) Streptomycin
b) Penicillin
c) Co-trimoxazole
d) Chloramphenicol

7. Bactericidal effect is:
a) Inhibition of bacterial cell division
b) Inhibition of young bacterial cell growth
c) Destroying of bacterial cells
d) Formation of bacterial L-form

8. Which of the following groups of antibiotics demonstrates a bactericidal effect?
a) Tetracyclines
b) Macrolides
c) Penicillins
d) All of the above

9. Bacteristatic effect is:
a) Inhibition of bacterial cell division
b) Inhibition of young bacterial cells growth
c) Destroying of bacterial cells
d) Formation of bacterial L-form

10. Which of the following groups of antibiotics demonstrates a bacteristatic effect:
a) Carbapenems
b) Macrolides
c) Aminoglycosides
d) Cephalosporins

11. Which of the following antibiotics contains a beta-lactam ring in their chemical structure :
a) Penicillins
b) Cephalosporins
c) Carbapenems and monobactams
d) All groups

12. Tick the drug belonging to antibiotics-macrolides:
a) Neomycin
b) Doxycycline
c) Erythromycin
d) Cefotaxime

13. Tick the drug belonging to antibiotics-carbapenems:
a) Aztreonam
b) Amoxacillin
c) Imipinem
d) Clarithromycin

14. Tick the drug belonging to antibiotics-monobactams:
a) Ampicillin
b) Bicillin-5
c) Aztreonam
d) Imipinem

15. Tick the drug belongs to antibiotics-cephalosporins:
a) Streptomycin
b) Cefaclor
c) Phenoxymethilpenicillin
d) Erythromycin

16. Tick the drug belonging to lincozamides:
a) Erythromycin
b) Lincomycin
c) Azithromycin
d) Aztreonam

17. Tick the drug belonging to antibiotics-tetracyclines:
a) Doxycycline
b) Streptomycin
c) Clarithromycin
d) Amoxacillin

18. All of antibiotics are aminoglycosides, EXCEPT:
a) Gentamycin
b) Streptomycin
c) Clindamycin
d) Neomycin

19. Tick the drug belonging to nitrobenzene derivative:
a) Clindamycin
b) Streptomycin
c) Azithromycin
d) Chloramphenicol

20. Tick the drug belonging to glycopeptides:
a) Vancomycin
b) Lincomycin
c) Neomycin
d) Carbenicillin

21. Antibiotics inhibiting the bacterial cell wall synthesis are:
a) Beta-lactam antibiotics
b) Tetracyclines
c) Aminoglycosides
d) Macrolides

22. Antibiotic inhibiting bacterial RNA synthesis is:
a) Erythromycin
b) Rifampin
c) Chloramphenicol
d) Imipinem

23. Antibiotics altering permeability of cell membranes are:
a) Glycopeptides
b) Polymyxins
c) Tetracyclines
d) Cephalosporins

24. All of the following antibiotics inhibit the protein synthesis in bacterial cells, EXCEPT:
a) Macrolides
b) Aminoglycosides
c) Glycopeptides
d) Tetracyclines

25. Biosynthetic penicillins are effective against:
a) Gram-positive and gram-negative cocci, Corynebacterium diphtheria, spirochetes, Clostridium gangrene
b) Corynebacterium diphtheria, mycobacteries
c) Gram positive cocci, viruses
d) Gram negative cocci, Rickettsia, mycotic infections

26. Which of the following drugs is a gastric acid resistant:
a) Penicillin G
b) Penicillin V
c) Carbenicillin
d) Procain penicillin

27. Which of the following drugs is penicillinase resistant:
a) Oxacillin
b) Amoxacillin
c) Bicillin-5
d) Penicillin G

28. All of the following drugs demonstrate a prolonged effect, EXCEPT:
a) Penicillin G
b) Procain penicillin
 c) Bicillin-1
d) Bicillin-5

29. Mechanism of penicillins' antibacterial effect is:
a) Inhibition of transpeptidation in the bacterial cell wall
b) Inhibition of beta-lactamase in the bacterial cell
c) Activation of endogenous proteases, that destroy bacterial cell wall
d) Activation of endogenous phospholipases, which leads to alteration of cell membrane permeability

30. Pick out the beta-lactamase inhibitor for co-administration with penicillins:
a) Clavulanic acid
b) Sulbactam
c) Tazobactam
d) All of the above

31. Cephalosporines are drugs of choice for treatment of:
a) Gram-positive microorganism infections
b) Gram-negative microorganism infections
c) Gram-negative and gram-positive microorganism infections, if penicillins have no effect
d) Only bacteroide infections

32. Carbapenems are effective against:
a) Gram-positive microorganisms

b) Gram-negative microorganisms
c) Only bacteroide infections
d) Broad-spectum

33. All of the following antibiotics are macrolides, EXCEPT:
a) Erythromycin
b) Clarithromycin
c) Lincomycin
d) Roxythromycin

34. Tetracyclins have following unwanted effects:
a) Irritation of gastrointestinal mucosa, phototoxicity
b) Hepatotoxicity, anti-anabolic effect
c) Dental hypoplasia, bone deformities
d) All of the above

35. Tick the drug belonging to antibiotics-aminoglycosides:
a) Erythromycin
b) Gentamycin
c) Vancomycin
d) Polymyxin

36. Aminoglycosides are effective against:
a) Gram positive microorganisms, anaerobic microorganisms, spirochetes
b) Broad-spectum, except Pseudomonas aeruginosa
c) Gram negative microorganisms, anaerobic microorganisms
d) Broad-spectum, except anaerobic microorganisms and viruses

37. Aminoglycosides have the following unwanted effects:
a) Pancytopenia
b) Hepatotoxicity
c) Ototoxicity, nephrotoxicity
d) Irritation of gastrointestinal mucosa

38. Choose the characteristics of chloramphenicol:
a) Broad-spectum. Demonstrates a bactericidal effect.
b) Influences the Gram-positive microorganisms. Demonstrates a bactericidal effect.
c) Influences the Gram-negative microorganisms. Demonstrates a bactericidal effect.
d) Broad-spectum. Demonstrates a bacteristatic effect.

39. Chloramphenicol has the following unwanted effects:
a) Nephrotoxicity
b) Pancytopenia
c) Hepatotoxicity
d) Ototoxicity

40. Choose the characteristics of lincozamides:
a) Broad-spectrum. Demonstrates a bactericidal effect.
b) Influence mainly the anaerobic organisms, Gram negative cocci.
c) Broad-spectrum. Demonstrates a bacteristatic effect.
d) Influence mainly the anaerobic organisms, Gram positive cocci.

41. Lincozamides have the following unwanted effect:
a) Nephrotoxicity
b) Cancerogenity
c) Pseudomembranous colitis
d) Irritation of respiratory organs

42. Choose the characteristics of vancomicin:
a) It is a glycopeptide, inhibits cell wall synthesis active only against Gram-negative bacteria
b) It is a glycopeptide, that alters permeability of cell membrane and is active against anaerobic bacteria
c) It is a beta-lactam antibiotic, inhibits cell wall synthesis active only against Pseudomonas aeruginosa
d) It is a glycopeptide, inhibits cell wall synthesis and is active only against Gram-positive bacteria.

43. Vancomicin has the following unwanted effects:
a) Pseudomembranous colitis
b) Hepatotoxicity
c) "Red neck" syndrome, phlebitis
d) All of the above

44. Which of the following drugs is used for systemic and deep mycotic infections treatment:
a) Co-trimoxazol
b) Griseofulvin
c) Amphotericin B
d) Nitrofungin

45. Which of the following drugs is used for dermatomycosis treatment:

a) Nystatin

b) Griseofulvin

c) Amphotericin B

d) Vancomycin

46. Which of the following drugs is used for candidiasis treatment:

a) Griseofulvin

b) Nitrofungin

c) Myconazol

d) Streptomycin

47. All of the following antifungal drugs are antibiotics, EXCEPT:

a) Amphotericin B

b) Nystatin

c) Myconazol

d) Griseofulvin

48. Mechanism of Amphotericin B action is:

a) Inhibition of cell wall synthesis

b) Inhibition of fungal protein synthesis

c) Inhibition of DNA synthesis

d) Alteration of cell membrane permeability

49. Azoles have an antifungal effect because of:

a) Inhibition of cell wall synthesis

b) Inhibition of fungal protein synthesis

c) Reduction of ergosterol synthesis

d) Inhibition of DNA synthesis

50. Which of the following drugs alters permeability of Candida cell membranes:

a) Amphotericin B

b) Ketoconazole

c) Nystatin

d) Terbinafine

51. Amfotericin B has the following unwanted effects:

a) Psychosis

b) Renal impairment, anemia

c) Hypertension, cardiac arrhythmia

d) Bone marrow toxicity

52. Tick the drug belonging to antibiotics having a polyene structure:
a) Nystatin
b) Ketoconazole
c) Griseofulvin
d) All of the above

53. All of the following drugs demonstrate a fungicidal effect, EXCEPT:
a) Terbinafin
b) Amfotericin B
c) Ketoconazole
d) Myconazol

54. Characteristics of polyenes are following, except:
a) Alter the structure and functions of cell membranes
b) Broad-spectrum
c) Fungicidal effect
d) Nephrotoxicity, hepatotoxicity

55. Characteristics of Amfotericin B are following, EXCEPT:
a) Used for systemic mycosis treatment
b) Poor absorption from the gastro-intestinal tract
c) Does not demonstrate nephrotoxicity
d) Influences the permeability of fungus cell membrane

Answer Key

01-B,02-D,03-B,04-D,05-B,06-C,07-C,08-C,09-A,10-B,11-D,12-C,13-C,14-C,15-B,16-B,17-A,18-C,19-D,20-A,21-A,22-B,23-B,24-C,25-A,26-B,27-A,28-A,29-A,30-D,31-C,32-D,33-C,34-D,35-B,36-D,37-C,38-A,39-B,40-D,41-C,42-D,43-C,44-C,45-B,46-C,47-C,48-D,49-C,50-C,51-B,52-A,53-B,54-C,55-C

38. Synthetic Antibacterial Drugs

1. Sulfonamides are effective against:
a) Bacteria and Chlamidia
b) Actinomyces
c) Protozoa
d) All of the above

2. Mechanism of sulfonamides' antibacterial effect is:
a) Inhibition of dihydropteroate reductase
b) Inhibition of dihydropteroate synthase
c) Inhibition of cyclooxygenase
d) Activation of DNA gyrase

3. Combination of sulfonamides with trimethoprim:
a) Decreases the unwanted effects of sulfonamides
b) Increases the antimicrobial activity
c) Decreases the antimicrobial activity
d) Increases the elimination of sulfonamides

4. Sulfonamide potency is decreased in case of co-administration with:
a) Oral hypoglycemic agents
b) Local anesthetics – derivatives of paraaminobenzoic acid
c) Local anesthetics – derivatives of benzoic acid
d) Non-narcotic analgesics

5. The following measures are necessary for prevention of sulfonamide precipitation and crystalluria:
a) Taking of drinks with acid pH
b) Taking of drinks with alkaline pH
c) Taking of saline drinks
d) Restriction of drinking

6. Resorptive sulfonamides have the following unwanted effects on blood system:
a) Hemolytic anemia
b) Thrombocytopenia
c) Granulocytopenia
d) All of the above

7. Mechanism of Trimethoprim' action is:
a) Inhibition of cyclooxygenase
b) Inhibition of dihydropteroate reductase
c) Inhibition of dihydropteroate synthase
d) Inhibition of DNA gyrase

8. Sulfonamides have the following unwanted effects:
a) Hematopoietic disturbances
b) Crystalluria
c) Nausea, vomiting and diarrhea
d) All of the above

9. Tick the drug, which is effective against mycobacteria only:
a) Isoniazid
b) Streptomycin
c) Rifampin
d) Kanamycin

10. Tick the antimycobacterial drug belonging to first-line agents:
a) PAS
b) Isoniazid
c) Kanamycin
d) Pyrazinamide

11. Tick the antimycobacterial drug, belonging to second-line agents:
a) Isoniazid
b) PAS
c) Rifampin
d) Streptomycin

12. Tick the antimycobacterial drug, belonging to antibiotics:
a) Isoniazid
b) PAS
c) Ethambutol
d) Rifampin

13. Tick the antimycobacterial drug – hydrazide of isonicotinic acid:
a) Rifampin
b) Isoniazid
c) Ethambutol
d) Pyrazinamide

14. Mechanism of Izoniazid action is:
a) Inhibition of protein synthesis
b) Inhibition of mycolic acids synthesis
c) Inhibition of RNA synthesis
d) Inhibition of ADP synthesis

15. Mechanism of Rifampin action is:
a) Inhibition of mycolic acids synthesis
b) Inhibition of DNA dependent RNA polymerase
c) Inhibition of topoisomerase II
d) Inhibition of cAMP synthesis

16. Mechanism of Cycloserine action is:
a) Inhibition of mycolic acids synthesis
b) Inhibition of RNA synthesis
c) Inhibition of cell wall synthesis
d) Inhibition of pyridoxalphosphate synthesis

17. Mechanism of Streptomycin action is:
a) Inhibition of cell wall synthesis
b) Inhibition of protein synthesis
c) Inhibition of RNA and DNA synthesis
d) Inhibition of cell membranes permeability

18. Rifampin has the following unwanted effect:
a) Dizziness, headache
b) Loss of hair
c) Flu-like syndrome, tubular necrosis
d) Hepatotoxicity

19. Isoniazid has following unwanted effect:
a) Cardiotoxicity
b) Hepatotoxicity, peripheral neuropathy
c) Loss of hair
d) Immunotoxicity

20. Ethambutol has the following unwanted effect:
a) Cardiotoxicity
b) Immunetoxicity
c) Retrobulbar neuritis with red-green color blindness
d) Hepatotoxicity

21. Streptomycin has the following unwanted effect:
a) Cardiotoxicity
b) Hepatotoxicity
c) Retrobulbar neuritis with red-green color blindness
d) Ototoxicity, nephrotoxicity

22. Mechanism of aminosalicylic acid action is:
a) Inhibition of mycolic acids synthesis
b) Inhibition of folate synthesis
c) Inhibition of DNA dependent RNA polymerase
d) Inhibition of DNA gyrase

23. All of the following agents are the first-line antimycobacterial drugs, EXCEPT:
a) Rifampin
b) Pyrazinamide
c) Isoniazid
d) Streptomycin

24. All of the following antimycobacterial drugs have a bactericidal effect, EXCEPT:
a) Pyrazinamide
b) Streptomycin
c) Rifampin
d) Isoniazid

25. Combined chemotherapy of tuberculosis is used to:
a) Decrease mycobacterium drug-resistance
b) Increase mycobacterium drug-resistance
c) Decrease the antimicrobal activity
d) Decrease the onset of antimycobacterial drugs biotransformation:

26. Tick the antibacterial drug – a nitrofurane derivative:
a) Nitrofurantoin
b) Trimethoprim
c) Ciprofloxacin
d) Nystatin

27. Tick the antibacterial drug – a nitroimidazole derivative:
a) Clavulanic acid
b) Metronidazole
c) Nitrofurantoin
d) Doxycycline

28. Tick the antibacterial drug – a quinolone derivative:
a) Nitrofurantoin
b) Nalidixic acid
c) Streptomycin
d) Metronidazole

29. Tick the antibacterial drug – a fluoroquinolone derivative:
a) Chloramphenicol
b) Nitrofurantoin
c) Nalidixic acid
d) Ciprofloxacin

30. Tick the indications for nitrofuranes:
a) Infections of respiratory tract
b) Infections of urinary and gastro-intestinal tracts
c) Syphilis
d) Tuberculosis

31. Tick the unwanted effects of nitrofuranes:
a) Nausea, vomiting
b) Allergic reactions
c) Hemolytic anemia
d) All of the above

32. Tick the indications for Metronidazole:
a) Intra-abdominal infections, vaginitis, enterocolitis
b) Pneumonia
c) As a disinfectant
d) Influenza

33. Tick the unwanted effects of Metronidazole:
a) Nausea, vomiting, diarrhea, stomatitis
b) Hypertension
c) Disturbances of peripheral blood circulation
d) All of the above

34. The mechanism of fluoroquinolones' action is:
a) Inhibition of phospholipase C
b) Inhibition of DNA gyrase
c) Inhibition of bacterial cell synthesis
d) Alteration of cell membrane permeability

35. Fluoroquinolones are active against:
a) Gram negative microorganisms only
b) Mycoplasmas and Chlamidiae only
c) Gram positive microorganisms only
d) Variety of Gram-negative and positive microorganisms, including Mycoplasmas and Chlamidiae

36. Tick the unwanted effects of fluoroquinolones:
a) Hallucinations
b) Headache, dizziness, insomnia
c) Hypertension
d) Immunetoxicity

37. Tick the indications for fluoroquinolones:
a) Infections of the urinary tract
b) Bacterial diarrhea
c) Infections of the urinary and respiratory tract, bacterial diarrhea
d) Respiratory tract infections

38. The drug of choice for syphilis treatment is:
a) Gentamycin
b) Penicillin
c) Chloramphenicol
d) Doxycycline

Answer Key

01-D,02-B,03-B,04-B,05-B,06-D,07-B,08-D,09-A,10-B,11-B,12-D,13-B,14-B,15-B,16-C,17-B,18-C,19-B,20-C,21-D,22-B,23-B,24-A,25-A,26-A,27-B,28-B,29-D,30-B,31-D,32A,33-A,34-B,35D,36-B,37-C,38-B

39. Antiprotozoal and anthelmintic Drugs

1. Tick the drug used for malaria chemoprophylaxis and treatment:
a) Chloroquine
b) Quinidine
c) Quinine
d) Sulfonamides

2. Tick the drug used for amoebiasis treatment:
a) Nitrofurantoin
b) Iodoquinol
c) Pyrazinamide
d) Mefloquine

3. Tick the drug used for trichomoniasis treatment:
a) Metronidazole
b) Suramin
c) Pyrimethamine
d) Tetracycline

4. Tick the drug used for toxoplasmosis treatment:
a) Chloroquine
b) Tetracyclin
c) Suramin
d) Pyrimethamine

5. Tick the drug used for balantidiasis treatment::
a) Azitromycin
b) Tetracycline
c) Quinine
d) Trimethoprim

6. Tick the drug used for leishmaniasis treatment:
a) Pyrimethamine
b) Albendazole
c) Sodium stibogluconate
d) Tinidazole

7. Tick the antimalarial drug belonging to 8-aminoquinoline derivatives:
a) Doxycycline
b) Quinidine
c) Primaquine
d) Chloroquine

8. All of the following antimalarial drugs are 4-quinoline derivatives, EXCEPT:
a) Chloroquine
b) Mefloquine
c) Primaquine
d) Amodiaquine

9. Tick the antimalarial drug belonging to pyrimidine derivatives:
a) Mefloquine
b) Pyrimethamine
c) Quinidine
d) Chloroquine

10. Tick the drug used for trypanosomosis treatment:
a) Melarsoprol
b) Metronidazole
c) Tetracyclin
d) Quinidine

11. Tick the antimalarial drug having a gametocidal effect:
a) Mefloquine
b) Primaquine
c) Doxycycline
d) Sulfonamides

12. All of the following antimalarial drugs influence blood schizonts, EXCEPT:
a) Mefloquine
b) Chloroquine
c) Primaquine
d) Quinidine

13. Tick the antimalarial drug influencing tissue schisonts:
a) Mefloquine
b) Chloroquine
c) Quinidine
d) Primaquine

14. Tick the group of antibiotics having an antimalarial effect:
a) Aminoglycosides
b) Tetracyclins
c) Carbapenems
d) Penicillins

15. Tick the amebecide drug for the treatment of an asymptomatic intestinal form of amebiasis:
a) Chloroquine
b) Diloxanide
c) Emetine
d) Doxycycline

16. Tick the drugs for the treatment of an intestinal form of amebiasis:
a) Metronidazole and diloxanide
b) Diloxanide and streptomycin
c) Diloxanide and Iodoquinol
d) Emetine and metronidazole

17. Tick the drug for the treatment of a hepatic form of amebiasis:
a) Diloxanide or iodoquinol
b) Tetracycline or doxycycline
c) Metronidazole or emetine
d) Erythromycin or azitromycin

18. Tick the luminal amebecide drug:
a) Metronidazole
b) Emetine
c) Doxycycline
d) Diloxanide

19. Tick the drug of choice for the treatment of extraluminal amebiasis:
a) Iodoquinol
b) Metronidazole
c) Diloxanide
d) Tetracycline

20. Tick the drug, blocking acetylcholine transmission at the myoneural junction of helminthes:
a) Levamisole

b) Mebendazole
c) Piperazine
d) Niclosamide

21. Tick niclosamide mechanism of action:
a) Increasing cell membrane permeability for calcium, resulting in paralysis, dislodgement and death of helminthes
b) Blocking acetylcholine transmission at the myoneural junction and paralysis of helminthes
c) Inhibiting microtubule synthesis in helminthes and irreversible impairment of glucose uptake
d) Inhibiting oxidative phosphorylation in some species of helminthes

22. Tick praziquantel mechanism of action:
a) Blocking acetylcholine transmission at the myoneural junction and paralysis of helminthes
b) Inhibiting microtubule synthesis in helminthes and irreversible impairment of glucose uptake
c) Increasing cell membrane permeability for calcium, resulting in paralysis, dislodgement and death of helminthes
d) Inhibiting oxidative phosphorylation in some species of helminthes

23. Tick piperazine mechanism of action:
a) Inhibiting microtubule synthesis in helminthes and irreversible impairment of glucose uptake
b) Blocking acetylcholine transmission at the myoneural junction and paralysis of helminthes
c) Inhibiting oxidative phosphorylation in some species of helminthes
d) Increasing cell membrane permeability for calcium, resulting in paralysis, dislodgement and death of helminthes

24. Tick the drug, a salicylamide derivative:
a) Praziquantel
b) Piperazine
c) Mebendazole
d) Niclosamide

25. Tick mebendazole mechanism of action:
a) Inhibiting oxidative phosphorylation in some species of helminthes
b) Increasing cell membrane permeability for calcium, resulting in paralysis, dislodgement and death of helminthes

c) Inhibiting microtubule synthesis in helminthes and irreversible impairment of glucose uptake

d) Blocking acetylcholine transmission at the myoneural junction and paralysis of helminthes

26. Tick the drug, inhibiting oxidative phosphorylation in some species of helminthes:
a) Niclosamide
b) Piperazine
c) Praziquantel
d) Mebendazole

27. Tick the drug for neurocysticercosis treatment:
a) Praziquantel
b) Pyrantel
c) Piperazine
d) Bithionol

28. Tick the drug for nematodosis (roundworm invasion) treatment:
a) Niclosamide
b) Praziquantel
c) Bithionol
d) Pyrantel

29. Tick the drug for cestodosis (tapeworm invasion) treatment:
a) Piperazine
b) Praziquantel
c) Pyrantel
d) Ivermectin

30. Tick the drug for trematodosis (fluke invasion) treatment:
a) Bithionol
b) Ivermectin
c) Pyrantel
d) Metronidazole

31. Tick the drug, a benzimidazole derivative:
a) Praziquantel
b) Mebendazole
c) Suramin
d) Pyrantel

32. Tick the broad spectrum drug for cestodosis, trematodosis and cycticercosis treatment:
a) Piperazine
b) Ivermectine
c) Praziquantel
d) Pyrantel

33. Tick the drug for ascaridosis and enterobiosis treatment:
a) Bithionol
b) Pyrantel
c) Praziquantel
d) Suramin

34. Tick the drug for strongiloidosis treatment:
a) Niclosamide
b) Praziquantel
c) Bithionol
d) Ivermectin

35. Tick the drug for echinococcosis treatment:
a) Suramin
b) Mebendazole or Albendazole
c) Piperazine
d) Iodoquinol

Answer Key

01-A,02-B,03-A,04-D,05-B,06-C,07-C,08-C,09-B,10-A,11-B,12-C,13-D,14-B,15-B,16-A,17-C,18-D,19-B,20-C,21-D,22-C,23-B,24-D,25-C,26-A,27-A,28-D,29-B,30-A,31-B,,32-C,33-B,34-D,35-B

40. Antiviral agents, Agents for Chemotherapy of Cancer

1. All of the following antiviral drugs are the analogs of nucleosides, EXCEPT:
a) Acyclovir
b) Zidovudine
c) Saquinavir
d) Didanozine

2. Tick the drug, a derivative of adamantane:
a) Didanozine
b) Rimantadine
c) Gancyclovir
d) Foscarnet

3. Tick the drug, a derivative of pyrophosphate:
a) Foscarnet
b) Zidovudine
c) Vidarabine
d) Acyclovir

4. Tick the drug, inhibiting viral DNA synthesis:
a) Interferon
b) Saquinavir
c) Amantadine
d) Acyclovir

5. Tick the drug, inhibiting uncoating of the viral RNA:
a) Vidarabine
b) Rimantadine
c) Acyclovir
d) Didanozine

6. Tick the drug, inhibiting viral reverse transcriptase:
a) Zidovudine
b) Vidarabine
c) Rimantadine
d) Gancyclovir

7. Tick the drug, inhibiting viral proteases:
a) Rimantadine
b) Acyclovir
c) Saquinavir
d) Zalcitabine

8. Tick the drug of choice for herpes and cytomegalovirus infection treatment:
a) Saquinavir
b) Interferon alfa
c) Didanozine
d) Acyclovir

9. Tick the drug which belongs to nonnucleoside reverse transcriptase inhibitors:
a) Zidovudine
b) Vidarabine
c) Nevirapine
d) Gancyclovir

10. All of the following antiviral drugs are antiretroviral agents, EXCEPT:
a) Acyclovir
b) Zidovudine
c) Zalcitabine
d) Didanozine

11. Tick the drug used for influenza A prevention:
a) Acyclovir
b) Rimantadine
c) Saquinavir
d) Foscarnet

12. Tick the drug used for HIV infection treatment, a derivative of nucleosides:
a) Acyclovir
b) Zidovudine
c) Gancyclovir
d) Trifluridine

13. Tick the antiviral drug which belongs to endogenous proteins:
a) Amantadine
b) Saquinavir
c) Interferon alfa
d) Pencyclovir

14. Tick the drug which belongs to nucleoside reverse transcriptase inhibitors:
a) Didanosine
b) Gancyclovir
c) Nevirapine
d) Vidarabine

15. All of the following antiviral drugs are anti-influenza agents, EXCEPT:
a) Acyclovir
b) Amantadine
c) Interferons
d) Rimantadine

16. Tick the unwanted effects of zidovudine:
a) Hallucinations, dizziness
b) Anemia, neutropenia, nausea, insomnia
c) Hypertension, vomiting
d) Peripheral neuropathy

17. Tick the unwanted effects of intravenous acyclovir infusion:
a) Renal insufficiency, tremors, delerium
b) Rash, diarrhea, nausea
c) Neuropathy, abdominal pain
d) Anemia, neutropenia, nausea, insomnia

18. Tick the drug that can induce peripheral neuropathy and oral ulceration:
a) Acyclovire
b) Zalcitabine
c) Zidovudine
d) Saquinavir

19. Tick the unwanted effects of didanozine:
a) Hallucinations, dizziness, insomnia
b) Anemia, neutropenia, nausea
c) Hypertension, vomiting, diarrhea
d) Peripheral neuropathy, pancreatitis, diarrhea, hyperuricemia

20. Tick the unwanted effects of indinavir:
a) Hypotension, vomiting, dizziness
b) Nephrolithiasis, nausea, hepatotoxicity
c) Peripheral neuropathy, pancreatitis, hyperuricemia
d) Anemia, neutropenia, nausea

21. Tick the drug that can induce nausea, diarrhea, abdominal pain and rhinitis:
a) Acyclovire
b) Zalcitabine
c) Zidovudine
d) Saquinavir

22. All of the following effects are disadvantages of anticancer drugs, EXCEPT:
a) Low selectivity to cancer cells
b) Depression of bone marrow
c) Depression of angiogenesis
d) Depression of immune system

23. Rational combination of anticancer drugs is used to:
a) Provide synergism resulting from the use of anticancer drugs with different mechanisms combination
b) Provide synergism resulting from the use of anticancer drugs with the same mechanisms combination
c) Provide stimulation of immune system
d) Provide stimulation of cell proliferation

24. Tick the anticancer alkylating drug, a derivative of chloroethylamine:
a) Methotrexate
b) Cisplatin
c) Cyclophosphamide
d) Carmustine

25. Tick the anticancer alkylating drug, a derivative of ethylenimine:
a) Mercaptopurine
b) Thiotepa
c) Chlorambucil
d) Procarbazine

26. Tick the group of hormonal drugs used for cancer treatment:
a) Mineralocorticoids and glucocorticoids
b) Glucocorticoids and gonadal hormones
c) Gonadal hormones and somatotropin
d) Insulin

27. Tick the anticancer alkylating drug, a derivative of alkylsulfonate:
a) Fluorouracil
b) Carboplatin
c) Vinblastine
d) Busulfan

28. Tick the anticancer drug of plant origin:
a) Dactinomycin
b) Vincristine
c) Methotrexate
d) Procarbazine

29. Action mechanism of alkylating agents is:
a) Producing carbonium ions altering protein structure
b) Producing carbonium ions altering DNA structure
c) Structural antagonism against purine and pyrimidine
d) Inhibition of DNA-dependent RNA synthesis

30. Tick the anticancer drug, a pyrimidine antagonist:
a) Fluorouracil
b) Mercaptopurine
c) Thioguanine
d) Methotrexate

31. Methotrexate is:
a) A purine antagonist
b) A folic acid antagonist
c) An antibiotic
d) An alkylating agent

32. Tick the antibiotic for cancer chemotherapy:
a) Cytarabine
b) Doxorubicin
c) Gentamycin
d) Etoposide

33. Fluorouracil belongs to:
a) Antibiotics
b) Antimetabolites
c) Plant alkaloids
d) Bone marrow growth factor

34. Tick the action mechanism of anticancer drugs belonging to plant alkaloids:
a) Inhibition of DNA-dependent RNA synthesis
b) Cross-linking of DNA
c) Mitotic arrest at a metaphase
d) Nonselective inhibition of aromatases

35. General contraindications for anticancer drugs are:
a) Depression of bone marrow
b) Acute infections
c) Severe hepatic and/or renal insufficiency
d) All of the above

36. Action mechanism of methotrexate is:
a) Inhibition of dihydrofolate reductase
b) Activation of cell differentiation
c) Catabolic depletion of serum asparagine
d) All of the above

37. Tick the anticancer drug belonging to inorganic metal complexes:
a) Dacarbazine
b) Cisplatin
c) Methotrexate
d) Vincristine

38. Tick the indication for estrogens in oncological practice:
a) Leukemia
b) Cancer of prostate
c) Endometrial cancer
d) Brain tumors

39. Enzyme drug used for acute leukemia treatment:
a) Dihydrofolate reductase
b) Asparaginase
c) Aromatase
d) DNA gyrase

40. All of the following drugs are derivatives of nitrosoureas, EXCEPT:
a) Carmustine
b) Vincristine
c) Lomustine
d) Semustine

41. Tick the group of drugs used as subsidiary medicines in cancer treatment:
a) Cytoprotectors
b) Bone marrow growth factors
c) Antimetastatic agents
d) All of the above

42. Tick the estrogen inhibitor:
a) Leuprolide
b) Tamoxifen
c) Flutamide
d) Anastrozole

43. Tick the antiandrogen drug:
a) Flutamide
b) Aminoglutethimide
c) Tamoxifen
d) Testosterone

44. Tick the drug belonging to aromatase inhibitors:
a) Octreotide
b) Anastrozole
c) Flutamide
d) Tamoxifen

45. Tick the drug belonging to gonadotropin-releasing hormone agonists:
a) Leuprolide
b) Tamoxifen
c) Flutamide
d) Anastrozole

Answer Key

01-C,02-B,03-A,04-D,05-B,06-A,07-C,08-D,09-C,10-A,11-B,12-B,13-C,14-A,14-A,16-B,17-A,18-B,19-D,20-B,21-D,22-C,23-A,24-C,25-B,26-B,27-D,28-B,29-B,30-A,31-B,32-B,33-B,34-C,35-D,36-A,37-B,38-B,39-A,40-B,40-D,42-B,43-A,44-B,45-A

Printed in Great Britain
by Amazon